OVERCOMING IMPOTENCE

A Doctor's Proven Guide to Regaining Sexual Vitality

STEVEN MORGANSTERN, M.D.
ALLEN ABRAHAMS, Ph.D.

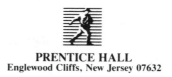

PRENTICE HALL
Englewood Cliffs, New Jersey 07632

Prentice-Hall International (UK) Limited, *London*
Prentice-Hall of Australia Pty. Limited, *Sydney*
Prentice-Hall Canada, Inc., *Toronto*
Prentice-Hall Hispanoamericana, S.A., *Mexico*
Prentice-Hall of India Private Limited, *New Delhi*
Prentice-Hall of Japan, Inc., *Tokyo*
Simon & Schuster Asia Pte. Ltd., *Singapore*
Editora Prentice-Hall do Brasil, Ltda., *Rio de Janeiro*

10 9 8 7 6 5 4 3 2

Library of Congress Cataloging-in-Publication Data

Morganstern, Steven
    [Love again, live again]
    Overcoming impotence : a doctor's proven guide to regaining sexual vitality /
Steven Morganstern and Allen Abrahams.
      p. cm.
    Rev. ed. of: Live again, love again. ©1988.
    Includes index.
    ISBN 0-13-146978-9
    1. Impotence—Popular works. I. Abrahams, Allan E. II. Morganstern,
Steven. Love again, live again. III. Title.
RC889.M758 1994
616.6'92—dc20   93-45909
                          CIP

ISBN 0-13-146960-6 NB2I
0-13-146978-9 (pbk)

PRENTICE HALL
Career and Personal Development
Englewood Cliffs, NJ 07632

Simon & Schuster, A Paramount Communications Company

Printed in the United States of America

How This Book Will Help You—And Your Partner

It is always rewarding to hear from the partners of men who have been successfully treated for sexual dysfunction. Susan did more than just send a short note. Instead, she wrote a detailed history of her husband's impotence problem, including how it nearly destroyed their marriage. She was thankful for the joyous change that took place after her husband obtained suitable professional treatment. In her letter, Susan expressed the hope that her experience would help other couples with similar problems. Near the beginning of the story, Susan recalled the following:

One evening, we met friends for dinner. With dinner Jesse had several drinks. While we were driving home, Jesse asked me why I had remained faithful to him. He could not understand why I did not have a lover. "I can't be a real husband to you when I'm only half a man."

Jesse and Susan were married in 1968, just twelve days after Jesse's return from Vietnam. About five years later, their marriage was a shambles, and a twelve-year period of "heartache, anxiety, and frustration" followed. In Susan's words:

Our lives became a turmoil of anger and hurt, misunderstanding and jealousy. Jesse became withdrawn and secretive; I became defensive and resentful. We seldom made love, and on the occasions when we did, it was totally unsuccessful—leaving us both empty and unfulfilled.

Regardless of all logic and constant reassurance, the typical impotence victim is convinced that he is somehow less than a man. "Being a man" in the sexual sense is important in our culture, and, for that matter, in virtually every culture. Despite frequent media ridicule of the excesses of "machismo," many American men, regardless of education, awareness, and sensitivity, equate successful sexual per-

iii

formance with maleness, self-worth, and the respect and even loyalty of their partners. Little can be done to convince them to the contrary. Fame, power, financial success, children, hobbies, or even a Nobel Prize provide little compensation.

Impotence is equally trying for the female partner. In a classic impotence pattern, Susan placed much of the blame on herself. She reasoned that she had become unattractive and, hence, undesirable to her husband. She had gained weight during the early years of their marriage, and she felt that perhaps this was the real cause of the trouble. Susan recalls feeling that her life was over: her children and work could not replace the void in her life.

Susan and Jesse's troubles eventually resulted in a two-year separation, although they later managed to reconcile. The eight years that followed were characterized by endless visits to marriage counselors, sex therapists, and health professionals, all of whom concluded that Jesse's problem was psychological in nature. None provided a workable solution. One even advised Susan to "dump" her husband while she was still young enough to start over.

Eventually, Jesse discovered that he had diabetes, a common cause of impotence. Susan recalls their almost perverse joy the day they learned that the underlying cause of their trouble was a potentially dangerous disease, rather than an emotional failing on their part. The diabetes, fortunately, could be controlled by diet. In contrast, implant surgery by a urologist was the only possible solution for Jesse's impotence problem.

Four weeks after surgery, Susan and Jesse successfully reconsummated their marriage. The long nightmare finally ended on the very day of their eighteenth wedding anniversary. Writing three months later, Susan reported some interesting changes in their life: the tension was gone, the children seemed happier, she felt prettier and was actively trying to lose weight, a coworker had commented to Jesse on how much easier he was to get along with.

The story of Jesse and Susan, as told here, first appeared in print in *Love Again, Live Again,* our first book on impotence and other forms of male sexual dysfunction (Prentice-Hall, 1988). Much has occurred in the interim. Today there are no longer any valid reasons for anybody to endure Jesse's and Susan's twelve-year nightmare. Impotence, or erectile dysfunction, is finally coming out of the closet, the final biological secrets of the male erection are unraveling, and more effective treatments are being reported almost routinely in the medical journals. Jesse and Susan and others who are willing to openly discuss their impotence problems deserve much of the credit.

Take the case of Alvin and Camille. During 1988, Jesse and Susan, along with the senior author, were asked to appear on a popular television talk show devoted to an hour-long discussion of all aspects of impotence. During the show, Jesse and Susan courageously shared their experiences with the large international electronic audience. The very next day Camille, who lived in Atlanta and had seen the program, called our offices at the nearby Morganstern Urology Clinic and set up an appointment for her husband, Alvin, age 42, who had been suffering from almost total impotence for the past six months. At our clinic, Alvin went through our standard initial patient interview and physical evaluation.

Alvin's impotence problem had seemed to first appear about six months earlier, just about the same time that he had started to take a drug of the beta blocker type for control of mild hypertension. The drug had been prescribed by Alvin's assigned HMO's "primary care provider," a physician whose specialty was gastroenterology. Alvin had complained to his physician about several problems that had seemed to have started after beginning to take the drug. These included, in addition to episodes of erectile failure, insomnia, difficulties in concentration, and depression. Alvin's physician never really responded to the impotence complaint. Instead, his advice was essentially limited to recommending a highly potent drug for treating the depression. He further scolded Alvin for having bothered to read the printed information on side effects that had accompanied the hypertension prescription, commenting that this type of material was "strictly for hypochondriacs."

We informed Alvin that the drug he had been taking had been definitely linked to impotence in some patients. We warned Alvin, however, that, due to the serious adverse health consequences of high blood pressure, he should continue for the moment to take this medication. At the same time, we referred Alvin to a highly regarded local cardiologist, with a known interest in hypertension. Alvin's impotence, along with the other side effects, vanished in a matter of days when he was prescribed a very effective alternate antihypertensive drug of the calcium channel blocker type.

Solving Alvin's problem was essentially a matter of the availability of good information, a suitable alternative drug, and proper medical concern. In the case of Roger, discussed next, the solution was the result of one of the very important advances in medical practice in recent years.

Roger, age 50, was referred to our office after his regular physician had reason to suspect the possibility of prostate cancer based upon a digital rectal examination performed during Roger's annual physical. Unfortunately, after suitable examination, we had to report to Roger that he did indeed have prostate cancer. Roger was initially devastated, not only because of the real threat to his life, but also because he was fully convinced that, at best, his sex life was over. It turned out that Roger had actually seen our television appearance about a year earlier, but the only thing that he could remember was our mentioning that prostate cancer often led to permanent impotence. He couldn't remember any of the things we also said regarding effective treatment.

It is a fact that only a few years ago, it was conventional wisdom that impotence was the highly likely outcome of all available surgical, radiation, or hormonal treatments of prostate cancer. Roger's impotence would have been dismissed as hopeless, but he would have been consoled with the advice that, after all, sex as you grow older was not all that important and impotence was certainly a small price to pay for the prolonging of life. Fortunately for Roger, this advice is no longer sound. In Roger's case, the cancer was promptly treated by radical prostectomy, the surgical removal of the entire prostate gland. Now about four years later, he has no sign of malignancy and should have many heathy years to come. He now also has a penile implant and is able to experience a totally fulfilling sexual life. In one of his periodic examinations, he summed it up as follows: "The next time I see you on television, Dr. Morganstern, I will listen a little more closely."

Despite increased open discussion of the impotence problem and advances in medical treatment, there still remains a downside. The percentage of the American adult male population subject to erectile difficulties appears to be even higher than previously suspected. Moreover, there is good reason to believe the total number of cases of impotence and other forms of male sexual dysfunction is rising. This is not only due to overall population increase and an aging American population, but also to such factors as the indiscriminate prescription of drugs for conditions such as hypertension and, all talk to the contrary, the declining quality of the American diet and the increasing number of men who fail to get proper exercise. Fortunately, should you be one of the rising number of men who experience impotence, there is no longer reason to accept your problem as an act of fate and unsolvable. Real hope exists for the majority of impotence sufferers, with effective treatment programs well within the budgetary limitations of most individuals.

The major purpose of this book is to make available a user-friendly and comprehensive information resource for men and their partners on all aspects of male sexual dysfunction. The emphasis throughout is on self-help: how to recognize whether a problem exists, where to get effective help, and how to choose between treatment options. It is hoped that the tools provided in this book will serve as a lifetime guide for your personal sexual fulfillment.

The first four chapters of this book provide useful and interesting background on the nature of impotence problems, including a description of how the male sexual mechanism should normally work, how it can malfunction, and the problems that can cause a malfunction. Chapter 5, which includes a very useful checklist and instructions for simple tests of your potency that you can perform in your home, will help you determine whether professional help is advisable. Chapter 6 provides information on where to best get help and what to expect, including a description of the tests usually performed by a urologist specializing in male sexual dysfunction.

Chapters 7 through 9 outline the various impotence treatment possibilities now available to help you choose the best treatment plan for your circumstance. Chapter 7 covers treatments based on hormones and drugs, while Chapter 8 covers the use of penile implants, reconstructive surgery, and external devices.

The role of psychotherapy and sex therapy in the treatment of impotence is examined in Chapter 9. Although it is now well recognized that at least 80 percent of all cases of impotence are due to physical causes and require physical solutions to be effective, psychotherapy and sex therapy can play a very important role in the successful restoration of sexual function in many patients. It is also recognized that psychotherapy and sex therapy can be very valuable in helping men and their partners deal with the serious emotional pain that typically accompanies impotence.

Chapter 10 covers the treatments of problems of male dysfunction, other than impotence. As the chapter indicates, troublesome problems, such as premature ejaculation, are finally yielding to modern medical treatment.

The ever-important question of how much treatment will cost is covered in Chapter 11. Important information is also given in the chapter regarding medical and hospital insurance and tax considerations. Chapter 12 deals with the prevention of impotence and how you can delay its onset if you are in a high-risk category. The chapter also includes some interesting examples of "impotence fraud" and tips on how to avoid being victimized by this unfortunately all-too-common problem.

Chapter 13 is addressed to Susan and to every other woman who shares in her partner's anguish. Useful advice is given the female partner as to how to cope with the emotional consequences of impotence from her perspective and ways to assist in the recommended program of treatment.

The final chapter, presented in question-and-answer form, serves as a general summary for the book and is intended to highlight the most common concerns typically voiced by men with sexual dysfunction problems. Additional useful information is given in the several appendices to the book, including a detailed listing of prescription and nonprescription drugs that have been linked to impotence, a suggested form for developing your relevant medical history, the names and addresses of support groups, a listing of drugs used to treat impotence and possible side effects, detailed advice on diet and exercise, and an extensive glossary.

Steven Morganstern, M.D.
Allen Abrahams, Ph.D.

Table of Contents

WHY IMPOTENCE IS MORE THAN A SEXUAL PROBLEM

The word "impotent" is used in common speech to describe a person of either gender lacking in power, strength, or vigor. At times, the meaning is broadened to imply the notion of helplessness. The word "impotence," as we will be using it, describes a familiar male sexual problem: a man who suffers from impotence is in some way incapable of normal sexual performance. Burdened with this condition, an impotent man has trouble enough without being told, or made to feel, that he is helpless. Nevertheless, the word that describes his medical problem does unfortunately carry quite negative connotations that challenge his very worth as a human being.

WHAT IS IMPOTENCE?

The word "impotence" is used very narrowly in this book to describe only a specific and usually medically treatable condition of a physical nature: the inability of a man to achieve and maintain an erection, adequate for vaginal penetration, to the mutual satisfaction of both parties. Impotence is completely unrelated to the character or manliness of the individual who suffers from this condition, and the sufferer must not ever try to take responsibility or "blame" for it.

When your car fails to start on a cold winter morning, you may become angry, and you may even blame yourself for not having had the car properly tuned in warmer weather, but to remedy the situation, you seek a mechanical solution; you do not blame the car! Similarly, this book emphasizes the physical nature of impotence and other problems of male sexual dysfunction and gives you scientific methods of diagnosis and treatment.

Impotence occurs in all men at one time or another. If the condition is experienced on a regular and persistent basis, it is referred to as chronic impotence and represents a medical problem that should never be ignored.

It is worth noting that in December 1992, a panel of experts convened under the auspices of the National Institutes of Health, a U.S. government entity in the medical field, recommended that the term "erectile dysfunction" be used in place of "impotence." The panel reasoned that the word "impotence" had serious negative implications; was used in an ambiguous manner; and, as a consequence, has contributed to confusing and uninterpretable results in both clinical and basic scientific investigations. There is much to be said for this recommendation. Nevertheless, throughout this book we have in most instances continued to use the word "impotence," despite its sometimes pejorative implications, reasoning that this is the term that is best known to the general public and, therefore, would be less confusing to our readers at the present time. In subsequent editions of this book, this usage could change.

It is not certain how many American males suffer from impotence and other forms of sexual dysfunction. Impotence is not a contagious disease, required by law to be reported to public health authorities. Part of the problem, as suggested already, is the ambiguous nature of the term and the difficulty of defining exactly when occasional impotence becomes regular and persistent. Another reason is that impotence victims have generally been "in the closet," usually too embarrassed to discuss their problems, even with their own physicians. Until quite recently, most American medical schools have regarded human sexuality in general, and especially male sexual dysfunction, as a taboo subject. In the past, the occasional researcher expressing interest in the field has often been viewed suspiciously by professional colleagues.

When was the last time, during an annual physical examination, that your doctor asked if you were experiencing any form of sexual dysfunction? If he or she has never asked you such a question, you have reason for concern. Bear in mind that sexual dysfunction is not only a problem in its own right, but can also be symptomatic of several serious underlying diseases.

WHY HEALTHY ERECTILE FUNCTION IS IMPORTANT

Impotence is admittedly an unpleasant condition, both for the victim and his partner, but it is seldom life threatening. People can live without sexual gratification. In fact, throughout history many men and women have taken vows of chastity, often for reasons of religious belief, and have still lived rich, fulfilling lives. Many people consider today's preoccupation with sex a failing of modern society and a cause of social ills. In addition, treatment for sexual dysfunction can be expensive, and in a world where many are hungry, it is often considered a personal indulgence. Nonetheless, there are several critical reason why impotence must always be dealt with:

1. Impotence and some other dysfunctions can prevent a man from fathering children.
2. Impotence strains family relationships.
3. Successful sexual performance indicates good health.
4. Impotence affects a man's job performance.
5. Sexual dysfunction can be linked to antisocial behavior.
6. Impotence is often a symptom of a serious underlying disease.
7. Impotence is a problem of particular concern to the elderly.

The Ability to Have Children

People have sex for procreational, recreational, and relational purposes. While some may deprecate the necessity of recreational sex in the family relationship, few fail to sympathize with the personal anguish of a financially secure and responsible young couple unable to have children. Widespread support appears to exist for the well-publicized in vitro or "test tube" approaches used in recent years to help infertile couples achieve pregnancy.

Failure to have children because of impotence places a very special emotional burden on the man. It is difficult enough for a man to be denied the pleasure of sexual intercourse and to fail to perform adequately as a lover. But the failure to have children because of impotence often makes the man feel that he has failed in his basic biological role to propagate the species. A man unable to have children due to some other problem, such as inadequate sperm count, may feel a sense of failure as well, but his guilt and self-loathing are inherently less than those of the man unable even to perform the act of sexual intercourse.

Treatment of impotence in childless couples can have very gratifying results. For example, consider the case of an impotent, 25-year-old, married patient who had suffered from diabetes since childhood. Because of religious beliefs, artificial insemination was not an option for him and his wife. Anguished and suicidal, he had already separated from his wife. Successful treatment included the implantation of an inflatable penile device. One year later, the man and his wife reconciled, and now they are the very happy parents of a baby girl.

It is important to understand that there is no special connection between impotence and male sterility. A male with an inadequate sperm count may be perfectly capable of engaging in normal intercourse. This, of course, is commonly the case with a man who has had a vasectomy. An impotent male, however, may have a normal sperm count. He may be able to father a child. This could be accomplished if the man were able to masturbate successfully to ejaculation, despite his inability to achieve an adequate erection for intercourse. The resulting ejaculate can be artificially inseminated into the female partner. This approach, however, is heroic in nature, it is potentially expensive, it has esthetic and psychological limitations, and it may be unacceptable because of a patient's religious beliefs.

Impotence is not the only condition in which male sexual dysfunction results in the inability to have children. Successful impregnation is obviously a problem in the case of premature ejaculation and the condition known as retro-grade ejaculation. In Peyronie's disease, the presence of scar tissue in the penis results in a bent erection, causing difficulty in achieving vaginal penetration and sometimes severe pain to both parties during intercourse. Other physical problems can make intercourse virtually impossible. Louis XVI of France, for many years, was unable to achieve penetration during intercourse with his wife, the notable Marie An-toinette, because of an exceptionally tight foreskin which prevented erection. The condition was surgically corrected, and the couple subsequently had children.

Impotence and Family Relationships

Impotence obviously exacts a severe toll on personal rela-tionships within the family. The condition often results in the man in fear, loss of self-image, and even potentially suicidal depression. The inner turmoil felt by the impotence sufferer may cause him to take his frustration out on his children and his wife, sometimes leading to the severing of family rela-tionships. Reliable statistical data do not exist to permit an analysis of the connection between the high national divorce rate and male sexual dysfunction. But sufficient evidence does exist, in the form of patients' comments, to suggest strongly that there is a connection.

Soap opera mentality provides the popular image of the oversexed, sexually dissatisfied, and unsympathetic wife who taunts her husband for his failures and seeks out the services of a readily available stud. This sometimes does occur, as was the case with John and Emily. John, 42 years old, had undergone coronary bypass surgery. As is often the case in men suffering with arterial disease, the condition extended to the genital area, resulting in his inability to perform sexually. Emily taunted John for his sexual failures and subsequently took a lover. John did not seek help for his sexual dysfunction and eventually died of a heart attack. The emotional strain of impotence and Emily's behavior may have been an important contributory factor in John's death.

Far more typical is the understanding and sympathetic woman, with normal sexual interests, driven to distraction by her partner's anguish and growing panic. In a typical scenario, the female partner may first respond with loving reassurance. As the condition persists, feelings of disappointment and resentment for the denial of pleasure and closeness may develop. The woman may gradually perceive her partner's problem as resulting from her lack of sexuality and physical desirability. Often the woman may suspect that the impotence is a consequence of her partner's active attention to another woman, which leaves him with little physical capacity to spare. Ultimately, the situation may deteriorate to total abstinence, expressions of anger and hostility, and finally, separation.

Personal Health

Impotence is not without its costs. In 1985, according to the National Hospital Discharge Survey conducted by the National Center for Health Statistics, impotence accounted for 30,000 hospital admissions and 400,000 outpatient visits to physicians. The direct cost of treatment at that time was reported at the $146 million level. The figure is obviously greater today given both rising population and inflating health care costs.

The indirect costs could be even greater. Male sexual dysfunction frequently goes hand in hand with the deteriorating physical and mental health of both of the involved partners, and even of other members of the family unit. A link between successful sexual performance and low incidence of certain diseases has been noted.

As the physical causes of impotence have become better appreciated, emphasis has shifted to its potentially very serious emotional consequences. Such consequences may include severe depression, hypochondria, insomnia, alcoholism, drug addiction, and suicide. Self-mutilation by despondent individuals has occurred on occasion.

It is not unusual for afflicted individuals, in desperation, to resort to quack cures, fad diets, gurus, and other assorted charlatans or to use potentially dangerous chemicals and bizarre mechanical devices. The historical neglect of dysfunction by responsible health care providers is a contributing factor to the widespread prevalence of these fake, and often dangerous, "cures." Zinc supplements, for example, have been heavily touted. A recent advertisement for a zinc supplement promised "bone hard erections." True to form, the advertisement showed the photograph of a smiling, obviously middle-aged man and an obviously ecstatic young woman. It is a fact that the mineral zinc plays a still not fully understood role in the functioning of the prostate gland; however, zinc deficiency in the United States is not a common problem, nor is there any scientific evidence that zinc supplements will cure erectile dysfunction.

At best, a person with a dysfunction may not be physically harmed by these approaches, although valuable time and money are usually lost. At worst, there can be serious consequences. In one recent case, a man had placed a "cock" ring around his penis in the hope that sufficient rigidity would be provided for intercourse. Use of the device, unfortunately, resulted in severe disfigurement. Numerous cases also exist in medical literature of patients who have placed rings and other devices around both the penis and the scrotum, necessitating surgical removal of the rings in hospital emergency rooms.

Job Productivity

Patients seeking treatment for sexual dysfunction often complain of difficulties in concentration, frequent mistakes, forgetfulness, impaired judgment, diminished creativity, and loss of drive. In extreme cases, dysfunction can lead to the psychological condition known as abulia, which results in the abnormal lack of ability to act or make decisions. Such conditions can easily result in lowered performance in the workplace, and sometimes even in termination of employment. For the university student suffering from these conditions, academic failure may result.

There is no way to put a price tag on the social cost of diminished worker productivity, but there is little doubt that the cumulative cost to the economy is substantial. Impotence seems to be widely distributed among all occupational groups. It has been suggested, however, that impotence is an especially common affliction among middle-level corporate managers who, as a group, are a major factor in the viability of the economic system. Such individuals are typically highly achievement oriented and competitive and, as a result, potentially very vulnerable when it comes to sexual failure.

It is possible only to speculate about the broader consequences of sexual dysfunction among individuals in critical occupations, such as the distracted airplane mechanic who forgets to install a vital component or the key public official suffering from a lack of concentration during a period of international crisis.

Antisocial Behavior

An all-too-frequent theme in the movies is the impotent man who is driven to commit some heinous crime out of frustration and anger because of his condition. Sometimes the plot revolves around the man who is capable of achieving erectile capability only while committing some horrible act of violence.

The fact is that such behavior is not common. It is more typical for the man suffering from erectile dysfunction to become passive and withdrawn. Nevertheless, there is some evidence that impotence may result in antisocial behavior in a small number of men with sometimes dire consequences. Nineteenth-century Russian anarchist Mikail Bakunin is principally remembered in history as a strident advocate of the violent overthrow of the existing social order. Over the years, many acts of terrorism were carried out by individuals influenced by the teachings of a man who had been labeled an "apostle of universal destruction." Bakunin's marriage is believed never to have been consummated, due to impotence.

Recent reports made available by the Russian KGB confirm longstanding rumors that Adolph Hitler had only one testicle. The reports are based upon autopsies performed by Red Army physicians on Hitler's body following the fall of Berlin. Might it be possible that Hitler suffered from a testosterone deficiency contributing to sexual failure? While not much is known about Hitler's sex life, it may be significant that he didn't marry until only a few hours before his death in the Berlin bunker. Some have suggested that Hitler's relationship with his consort, Eva Braun, may have been platonic in nature. In any event, Hitler never had children and apparently had very limited contact with women.

Sexual release is known to have a calming effect on male aggression. It is an open secret that prison officials often encourage situational homosexual behavior. In some more enlightened prisons, conjugal visits are permitted, not only to achieve a more docile convict population, but also as an aid to rehabilitation. Sexual dysfunction has been suggested as a factor in pederasty, the sexual abuse of children. The pederast, almost always a man, often suffers from performance anxiety. Sex with an adult partner, with normal sexual expectations, could result in great embarrassment were failure to occur. The pederast, therefore, turns to children, where such expectations do not exist, or where the victims may even be too young to understand the nature of the activity.

Obviously, not all men suffering from dysfunction have the evil potential of a Bakunin or a Hitler, or commit acts of child abuse. It is reasonable to suggest, however, that failure to treat afflicted individuals properly could, on occasion, have very serious social consequences.

Disease Symptoms

Impotence is a medical disorder characterized by the loss of a bodily function. The loss of any type of bodily function is not a normal occurrence and should be regarded as a sign or symptom of some underlying and possibly very serious medical condition. For this reason, no thorough physical examination of a patient is complete without systematic inquiry into the matter of sexual performance. Unfortunately, this is not often the case.

Good medical practice mandates the careful examination of a patient reporting impotence symptoms, especially for possible diabetic and cardiovascular problems. Diabetes mellitus is a serious disease characterized by the failure of the pancreas to secrete a sufficient quantity of the hormone insulin to allow for the proper absorption of glucose, a sugar critical in providing for the body's energy needs. Type I diabetes is largely a disease of children and has noticeable symptoms that develop over a short period of time. Obviously, impotence is rarely one of the symptoms of Type I diabetes. Type II diabetes, which may develop in men in their young and middle adult years, is another story. Often the symptoms are slow to appear and are not obvious in nature.

Early treatment is important, and impotence may be the first real sign that Type II diabetes exists.

Vascular disorders are a frequent factor underlying much erectile dysfunction. Problems in the vascular system are often silent in nature and may not be apparent until there is some life-threatening event. It is reasonable to suspect that when vascular deterioration is taking place in the penis, an organ along the periphery of the body, it could also be taking place at critical points elsewhere. Promptly paying heed to the impotence warning might save some patients from possible heart attack or stroke.

Even when impotence can be ultimately linked to psychological factors, prompt investigation of the initial symptoms has been well justified, since the underlying psychological causes are best identified and treated as early as possible.

Impotence and the Elderly

A tee shirt seen at a senior center bore the words "Dirty Old Men Need Loving Too." The sexual needs of the elderly are something that many of us don't like to discuss or even admit exist. The fact is that many older men and women still experience sexual interest and benefit from intimate relationships. There is evidence that older men are particularly sensitive to the social support of such relationships. The following is a typical situation faced by the elderly:

Henry at age 76 becomes a widower after 55 years of marriage. For about ten years prior to his wife's death, Henry had been experiencing erectile difficulties, but the very close couple had generally resolved the problem by touching and mutual masturbation. Henry's initial period of grief then leads to a subsequent period of loneliness and depression, during which his overall health begins to deteriorate. In the retirement community where Henry lives there are many suitable older women and he yearns for their company. He is afraid to approach any of them fearing that in the event a sexual relationship were to be called for, he would be sure to experience embarrassing sexual failure and, even worse, a painful incident of rejection.

Henry's fear of what might happen were he to get involved has further consequences. As women tend to live longer than men, women desiring companionship usually find few men available and therefore also suffer from the pain of loneliness. The shortage is compounded by reluctant men like Henry. There could very well be many women out there who would be understanding and sympathetic to Henry's impotence problem, or are primarily interested in companionship, rather than just dramatic sex, but Henry may never find out.

With a growing senior population, the problem of impotence in the elderly will not go away. As all of us sooner or later will grow old, it is not unreasonable to look for solutions that will make our senior years rewarding.

HOW MANY MEN ARE IMPOTENT?

If you are being treated for hypertension, there is a possibility that you will become impotent. High blood pressure is a serious medical problem that has received increasing attention in recent years. However, the drug or combination of drugs used to treat hypertension may contribute to impotence. Good medical practice should include a detailed profile of a patient's past sexual performance prior to the start of any treatment. The physician should warn the patient about the side effects of all drugs prescribed, especially those that have been linked to impotence. After treatment is underway, the patient should be closely monitored, and any impotence symptoms must be recorded. Unfortunately, all too often the question of impotence is never discussed unless it is brought up by an aggressive and knowledgeable patient.

Until very recently, there has been very little scientific research into the incidence of male sexual dysfunction, contributing to a lack of reliable statistical data on the problem. This is not surprising as human sexuality, in general, only began to appear as a required course in the curriculum of most medical schools during the past three decades, ironically at about the same time courses in sex education became common for school children. During the 1980s, Dr. William Looms Furlow, of the Mayo Clinic, estimated the number of American men experiencing chronic impotence (as of 1985) conservatively at 10 million. Given the number of men age 18 years or older at that time, it followed that roughly 12 percent of all American men were impotent. Furlow based his estimate on the number of men subject to various health problems that are closely linked to impotence, including diabetes, various vascular diseases, radical pelvic surgery, multiple sclerosis, and spinal cord injuries, plus an allowance for the probable number of men afflicted with impotence of a physiological nature. Many authorities at the time believed that the Furlow estimate was, while a good start, probably too conservative.

In mid-1992, the results of the Massachusetts Male Aging Study became available. This important study, conducted by researchers at the Department of Urology, Boston University, and the New England Research Institute, under a grant from the National Institutes of Health, was based upon an actual random sample of men, aged 40 to 70, living in the Boston area. The results of the study painted a far more disturbing picture: the combined prevalence of minimal, moderate, and complete impotence among the men was at the 52 percent level. In the study, of men who related themselves as just minimally impotent, 17.2 percent of those surveyed had trouble getting an erection 50 percent of the time and 63 percent of the time had a problem in sustaining the erection and keeping it for sufficient length of time. The 9.6 percent of the men who rated themselves as completely impotent had trouble getting an erection 90 percent of the time and keeping it 96 percent of the time. The largest number of men, 25.2 percent, fell into the moderately impotent category. In this group, a problem existed in getting an erection 85 percent of the time and keeping it 95 percent of the time.

On the basis of the statistical analysis, the researchers concluded that some degree of impotence is present in 30 million American men, three times the Furlow estimate. The researchers also found a close association of impotence with age, reporting that complete impotence tripled between ages 40 and 70.

Unless there is just something wrong with Boston men, a highly unlikely proposition, the implications of the Massachusetts study are staggering. Given the current number of American males, the 30 million figure just cited would suggest that possibly as many as three out of eight American men are impotent. The next time you are in a large group of men, perhaps on the job or at a sports event, glance around. It may be some small consolation, if you suffer from impotence, to know you are not alone.

Little is known about the prevalence of impotence in the male population as it relates to such characteristics as ethnic origin, race, and socioeconomic group. Impotence affects individuals in all walks of life. Some public figures reported to have suffered from erectile dysfunction, in addition to those previously mentioned, include Dwight David Eisenhower, Chinese Emperor P'u-Yi, and John Ruskin. Eisenhower is believed to have had a close relationship with his driver, Kay Summersby, while serving as Supreme Allied Commander in Europe during World War II. The relationship is said to have never been consummated, due to an impotence problem. Significantly, Eisenhower suffered from serious cardiovascular problems while serving as the thirty-fourth president of the United States.

P'u-Yi assumed his throne as an infant. His pathetic life story was the subject of the excellent movie *The Last Emperor*. In later life, as a prisoner, he suffered humiliation at the hands of Communist leader Mao Tse-tung over his problem. The marriage of John Ruskin, prominent nineteenth-century British writer and social critic, was never consummated. Ruskin is known to have had a history of bad health, including evidence of vascular disorder.

One thing that is quite certain is that there is little evidence to support popular stereotypes as to the sexual prowess of members of certain races and ethnic groups. Woody Allen, in his hilarious movie, *Sleeper,* depicts a world of the future in which both males and females have lost their sexual powers. Allen's characters had to seek sexual gratification by the use of a mechanical device suggestive of an old-time telephone booth. In Allen's movie, only men of Italian ethnic origin retained their sexual prowess. With all due respect to the Italian stallions among us, this ethnic stereotype has yet to be proven by valid scientific investigation.

Similar stereotypes exist, of course, with respect to African Americans and Hispanics. African-American and Hispanic men, nevertheless, frequently turn up at urologists' offices or at impotence support group meetings. It is reasonable to suspect that many of these men bear the additional psychological burden of living up to popular ethnic expectations, as well as the emotional anguish of their underlying condition. Actually, impotence could very well be disproportionately present in both the African-American and Hispanic communities. In the case of the former, hypertension constitutes a very common problem, and there is also the problem of sickle-cell anemia. In the case of the latter, diabetes is very common.

Very little is known about the incidence of impotence and other male sexual dysfunction problems outside the United States. Third World countries such as Mexico, Brazil, Nigeria, and India are characterized by relatively young populations, which would presumably imply a lower incidence of impotence. On the other hand, health conditions in these countries and the high popularity of cigarette smoking could take its toll. The situation in the advanced industrial countries of the European Community and Japan is probably similar to that in the United States. The Japanese, and other Asians, eat a better diet than do Americans in terms of cholesterol, a factor in heart disease and hypertension and erectile dysfunction, but the benefits could be canceled out by almost universal smoking by adult men. Preliminary reports out of Russia available to the authors indicate the possibility of high levels of impotence in the former Soviet Union and Eastern Europe. Poor diet, cigarette smoking, and excessive consumption of alcohol are all serious problems in these countries.

IS IMPOTENCE MORE COMMON TODAY?

A very interesting question is whether impotence and other forms of male sexual dysfunction are becoming more common in the American population. A very popular belief is that the emergence during the late 1960s of the feminist movement and the "new woman" resulted in an increase in performance anxiety and other psychological factors. There is, however, virtually no tangible scientific evidence to support this view. In addition, there is virtually no reliable information available on the long-term incidence of impotence in the American population. A case might be made, incidentally, that the advent of the more aware and assertive woman has contributed to a situation where there is greater willingness to confront and deal with the impotence problem.

Several trends, all related to physical rather than psychological causes, however, suggest the strong possibility of a growing impotence problem. One trend is the aging demographic profile of the U.S. population. With the U.S. population growing at a relatively low rate, and the reduced birth rates of recent years, a greater percentage of the male population is now concentrated in the higher age brackets. As demonstrated in the Massachusetts Male Aging Study, age is the single variable most often associated with impotence. A second factor is the increasing public awareness and concern about high blood pressure, combined with the often indiscriminate prescription of antihypertensive drugs that can lead to impotence. Finally, impotence can be associated with various forms of drug abuse, including tobacco, cocaine and crack, and excessive consumption of alcohol, all of which remain prevalent in our society.

The burden is clearly on the individual sufferer and his partner to take charge to obtain proper treatment for male sexual dysfunction. The more knowledgeable the sufferer is, the more aggressive and successful he will be in obtaining proper treatment. Unfortunately, public attitudes and lack of knowledge about the impotence problem are still appalling.

According to a survey conducted on behalf of the Impotence Information Center and released in 1986, nearly one-half of the general public was reluctant even to discuss the subject, with such reluctance increasing with age. Of those who were willing to consider the subject, about 45 percent were unable to name a single physical cause of impotence, and 90 percent were totally unaware of the very important diabetes-impotence link. A large segment of the population was unable to define impotence properly, many confused the concept with infertility, and most were unable to identify the medical specialists who provide treatment.

Impotence sufferers presumably can be expected to be more knowledgeable about the subject. Nevertheless it is believed that less than 5 percent of men with the problem seek medical treatment, which, if true, might make impotence the most common untreated medical disorder. It is still not at all uncommon to encounter male patients who have waited many years before seeking treatment. Such individuals have endured personal tragedy that approaches martyrdom for a condition that, in their ignorance, they tend to blame on themselves.

Fortunately, such attitudes may soon be in the past. Evidence of growing knowledge and awareness include the overwhelming response by telephone and mail to our numerous appearances on television and radio talk shows; the number of inquiries received by the Impotence Information Center, the Impotence Institute, and other information sources; and increased attendance at meetings of the support group Impotents Anonymous. As this book itself demonstrates, there is now a wealth of practical information available. Prior to the mid-1980s, very little was available except that expressed in highly technical terms in the medical journals.

Impotence is more than just a sexual problem. Given the importance of male sexuality and potentially serious consequences of impotence, it is a problem that always should be promptly medically investigated and treated in an appropriate manner. Just because impotence is associated with aging, there is no reason to be fatalistic and do nothing about the problem. Declining vision is also part of the aging process, but that is no excuse for not getting eyeglasses. Effective and affordable help is now available for those willing to actively seek assistance.

CHAPTER 2

IMPOTENCE IN HISTORICAL PERSPECTIVE

Despite the great advances that have been made in recent years in understanding the causes of impotence and other male sexual problems, many incorrect beliefs of the past discourage men from seeking treatment and continue to impact unfavorably on treatment programs. It is helpful for men with impotence problems, and their partners, to become familiar with past beliefs and treatment approaches, in order to be on guard for the possible persistence of antiquated attitudes even among health care professionals.

ANCIENT BELIEFS

Erectile dysfunction has been a problem since the dawn of history. The ancients typically attributed such problems to the wrath of the gods or the use of witchcraft by enemies. Treatment involved placating the gods with appropriate offerings, or using aphrodisiacs, magic, and the occult.

An Old Testament story (Genesis 20:1-18) has been interpreted as telling of how Abimelech, due to divine intervention, was rendered incapable of successful sexual performance. The minor tribal king's problem had developed following his abduction of Sarah, the wife of the patriarch Abraham. The story fortunately has a happy ending, as Abimelech's full powers were restored with the release of Sarah and with the prayers on Abimelech's behalf by, of all people, the wronged husband.

Impotence was considered by the ancients a fatal flaw in a ruler. David was deposed as king of Israel when he "knew her not," after his courtiers had provided the services of the young virgin, Abishag the Shumanite, in an abortive attempt to restore the vigor of the aged monarch (First Kings 1:1-34). This attitude still persists in some countries with a Latin tradition. It is an asset to a politician to be known for his frequent and varied sexual accomplishments.

Among the ancient Greeks, it was a common belief that impotence would ultimately be experienced by any man who had been placed on top of a tomb as a child. One possible cure was to take a noxious potion based on the scrapings from the blade of a knife used for gelding rams.

To this day, men still pray to the gods. In Japan, a certain religious shrine is dedicated to male sexual problems. Japanese men, in traditional dress, regularly gather around a large erect wooden penis and seek the help of Shinto deities. Magic potions are still very much in vogue. While on a visit several years ago to Bahia, Brazil, one of the authors was shown, by a high priestess of the African-derived macumba cult, a selection of fearsome-looking preparations suitable for curing impotence. According to the priestess, requests for impotence remedies are about as common as requests for potions to cure intestinal parasites and were often made by wealthy and highly educated individuals.

ATTITUDES OF NINETEENTH-CENTURY MEDICINE

By the nineteenth century, medical science had advanced to the point that a scientific approach to impotence was possible. In fact, as early as the sixteenth century, Varolio, an Italian physician, had observed that the existence of an erection was related to the flow of blood through the penis. Despite great progress in medicine, in general, during the nineteenth century the treatment of male sexual dysfunction in many ways actually regressed.

The lack of progress can be linked to the highly prudish attitudes toward sex that prevailed during the Victorian era, with such attitudes typified by the use of the word "limbs" instead of "legs" and the strategic placement of fabrics to hide the apparently sexually suggestive legs of tables and chairs. In the supercharged moralistic environment of that period, it was inevitable that the medical establishment would find a connection between impotence and immoral activities, especially masturbation.

A classical statement of the approach of nineteenth-century medicine to the impotence problem appears in a fascinating promotional booklet published by Dr. T. W. Hughes, a licensed physician and surgeon practicing in Atlanta, Georgia, as late as 1926. The 72-page booklet, entitled *New Street Guide of Atlanta and Useful Medical Receipts*, contains, in addition to a street guide, valuable information on the removal of warts, glowing testimonials to Dr. Hughes, and comments on various medical problems, principally those of a sexual nature. In the exact words of Dr. Hughes, and keeping the original bold type, the passage reads as follows:

> *The causes of* **Sexual impotency,** *are as follows:* **Youthful Follies, Pollutions (night losses), Spermatorrhoea, Prostate Congestion, Gonorrhoea, Stricture, Narrow Meatus** *and many* **Organic Troubles,** *such as wasting of the* **Testicles, Variciele, Disobedience of Nature's Laws, Sexual Excess or Long Abstinence. Sedentary Habits, Worry, Anxiety and Business Cares,** *all tend to produce this end,* **rendering men powerless and devoid of natural function before their time.**

The term "Youthful Follies," of course, refers to masturbation or "self-abuse." "Pollutions" is a condition characterized by the "too frequent" occurrence of nocturnal emissions. There is, unfortunately, no explanation provided as to the meaning of the term "Disobedience of Nature's Laws."

The treatment of impotence by the nineteenth-century medical establishment was essentially limited to the crusade against masturbation and other moral abominations. Significantly, there is little evidence of any scientific attempt among nineteenth-century physicians to define the actual physical connection between masturbation and impotence. Means for dealing with the problem during the period included such advice as the avoidance of "bad thoughts" and the use of devices by young boys that discouraged the touching of the penis. Even in China today, men are advised not to sleep facing down, given the opportunity in this position to stimulate the penis.

Masturbation, incidentally, was blamed for more than just impotence. Among other things, it was the root cause of pollutions. Dr. Hughes would have you believe that boys who masturbate "have a sheepish, hang-dog expression" and "incline to melancholy broodings." Moreover, "their palms are apt to be cold and moist." Adult males who masturbate "are apt to be cowardly, mean-spirited poor specimens of humanity."

It would be a mistake to dismiss these attitudes as merely a nostalgic remembrance of a bygone era. It was only in 1948 that the Boy Scouts of America dropped the famous passage on the evils of masturbation from the pages of their official handbook. Masturbation can still get you into trouble if you are a member of the U.S. armed forces and get caught. Many older men who are today experiencing sexual dysfunction suffer from a residual burden of guilt extending back to exposure to these attitudes in childhood. It is not unreasonable to suspect that many physicians practicing today are still subject to such influences.

TRADITIONAL PSYCHOTHERAPY

The end of the nineteenth century saw the inevitable reaction to prevailing attitudes toward sex in the work of Sigmund Freud and various associates. Impotence, of course, figures in Freudian thought and is closely related to infantile sexuality, a key element in the Freudian scheme of things. A concise statement of Freud's approach to impotence appeared in an essay on "the Universal Tendency to Debasement in the Sphere of Love," published in 1912. In this essay, Freud commented that, following any forms of anxiety, "psychical" impotence was the most common disorder encountered in psychoanalytical practice. He further noted that the condition could be found in men of a strongly "libidinous" nature and in men who appear to have no physical condition that should prevent successful sexual performance.

According to Freud, the explanation for this is the "inhibitory influence of certain psychical complexes." Such complexes are not found in the conscious mind and, hence, are not apparent to the individual with the impotence problem. Of the possible complexes, none is more serious than an unresolved incestuous fixation on a mother or perhaps a sister dating back to childhood, in short, the Oedipus complex. Lesser complexes result from traumatic infantile sexual experiences, for example, the shame of a young boy who had been caught in an act of masturbation.

The traditional Freudian approach to the treatment of impotence, in essence, is no different from the treatment of any other inhibiting "psychical," that is, psychological, complex, the now-familiar process of psychoanalysis. In psychoanalysis, or the "talking cure," various childhood memories associated with the inhibiting complexes are gradually recalled from memory in extended sessions between the patient and the therapist. Somehow, an awareness of such memories results in the resolution of the complex, along with the eventual disappearance of any related physical and emotional problems.

In a relatively short period of time, traditional Freudian psychoanalysis would fragment into a spectrum of contentious and often pseudoscientific cults. Wide variations in treatment approaches also emerged, ranging from group therapy to hypnotherapy to primal scream therapy. It was increasingly acknowledged by all but the strictest followers of classical Freudian dogma that factors other than just those associated with incest and infant sexuality might result in impotence and other problems. At the same time, the idea that impotence was essentially "all in the head" became a fixed belief, not only among psychotherapists, but also throughout the general medical establishment. Little scientific interest was shown in the possible biological mechanisms by which problems "in the head" somehow resulted in a lack of physical performance in the penis.

By 1927, Wilhelm Stekel, a prominent European neuropsychiatrist and psychotherapist, was able to claim that practically all cases of impotence were linked to psychic inhibitions that could be treated with psychotherapy. Moreover, Stekel went on to theorize that underlying the psychic inhibitions resulting in impotence are various cultural forces such as religion, the family, and the political and economic systems. Such views, unfortunately, are at odds with the obvious existence of many sexually capable men in the most restrictive segments of modern society and the frequent discovery of impotent men in primitive societies where there are no restrictive institutions.

Wilhelm Reich, a former pupil of Freud, took the idea of psychic inhibitions past the edge, claiming that sexual repression was the major cause not only of sexual dysfunction but also neurosis, disease, and virtually every other problem known to humanity. The once-respected psychiatrist ended up in prison when he violated a court order obtained by the U.S. Food and Drug Administration and continued to promote the sale of a boxlike device known as an "orgone accumulator" as a potency stimulator and a cure for cancer. According to Reich, his device served to concentrate a form of energy, known as "orgone," a force associated with the orgasm and extending throughout the universe. Physical scientists have yet to confirm the reality of orgone.

Despite increasing evidence of the shortcomings of the "all-in-the-head" theories, David Reuben, M.D., in 1969 could still categorically state in his highly successful bestseller, *Everything You Always Wanted to Know About Sex but Were Afraid to Ask:* "There is a convincing evidence that the source of male potency is in the brain."[1] Reuben went on to acknowledge, however, that about 5 percent of all impotence has a physical basis. As to a possible cure for an impotence problem, Reuben suggested only psychiatry and hypnosis.

---

1 David R. Reuben, *Everything You Always Wanted to Know About Sex but Were Afraid to Ask* (New York: David McKay, 1969), pp. 98-99.

Surprisingly, *The Columbia University College of Physicians and Surgeons Complete Home Medical Guide,* a book aggressively promoted to the general public, in discussing impotence could still state in 1989: "In some men, the problem is caused by a disease, such as diabetes, or the result of prostate and other surgery. More often, however, the problem is psychological rather than physiological."[2]

Fortunately, there is evidence of growing understanding on the part of the medical establishment. In 1992, *The Johns Hopkins Medical Handbook,* after noting that only a decade earlier more than 90 percent of all impotence cases could be blamed on emotional causes, could add: "During the past 10 years, however, doctors have come to believe that at least half and perhaps as many as three quarters of all cases have a physiological basis as well."[3]

THE ERA OF SEX THERAPY

Until very recently, the subject of human sexuality received short shrift at most medical schools and in the general scientific community. The problem of impotence in particular was not investigated from a medical viewpoint. Those researchers who did study sexuality were wedded to traditional psychoanalytical approaches, which prevented them from conducting systematic scientific investigations.

In 1922, the results of research over the years by William H. Masters, M.D., Virginia E. Johnson, and others at the

2 Donald F. Tapley et al., *The Columbia University College of Physicians and Surgeons Complete Home Medical Guide,* rev. ed. (New York: Crown, 1989), p.181.
3 Simeon Margolis and Hamilton Moses III, *The Johns Hopkins Medical Handbook* (New York: Rebus, 1992), p.396.

Reproductive Biology Research Foundation, St. Louis, Missouri, appeared in the book *Human Sexual Response*.[4] Despite the highly technical nature of the findings, the book caused an immediate sensation. Unfortunately, an undeniable factor in the book's success was the public's titillation with the experimental methods employed in the research project, such as direct observation of the actual sexual performance of male and female volunteers and the use of cameras, cardiographs, blood monitors, and other laboratory devices. In 1970, Masters and Johnson followed up with a second book, *Human Sexual Inadequacy,* which dealt specifically with problems of sexual dysfunction in both males and females. This time the public was treated to reports of the use of sexual "surrogates" in the experimental program.[5]

The Masters and Johnson studies must be regarded as a major milestone in the understanding of how erotic stimulation impacts on the human body anatomically and physiologically. They have also provided some very valuable information on sexual dysfunction. On the other hand, the studies have tended to perpetuate the traditional belief that impotence is essentially a psychological problem. It is important to observe, however, that the original Masters and Johnson studies concede the possibility of physical causes of impotence, at least in some cases.

A key belief in the Masters and Johnson system is that a variety of psychological stress factors result in impotence. "Performance anxiety," or the excessive fear of the consequences of unsuccessful sexual performance, is singled out as being especially important. Performance anxiety, more-

4 William H. Masters and Virginia E. Johnson, *Human Sexual Response* (Boston: Little, Brown, 1966).
5 William H. Masters and Virginia E. Johnson, *Human Sexual Inadequacy* (Boston: Little, Brown, 1970).

over, is believed to be self-reinforcing, with episodes of failure resulting in cycles of heightened anxiety and repeated failure.

The Masters and Johnson studies, however, provided little insight into the actual mechanism at work within the human body by which fears and anxieties centered in the brain result in the loss of erection. Some observers have suggested that performance anxiety could trigger surges of the chemical epinephrine, better known as adrenalin, into the bloodstream. This, in turn, could result in a diminished flow of blood to the penis and loss of erection.

Treatment methods based on the Masters and Johnson theories of sexual dysfunction typically involve an active approach, which ranges from masturbation exercises to participation by the sexual partners in various exercises in touching, fondling, and so forth. This approach has been labeled sensate focus therapy. The emphasis in "sensate focus" therapy is on direct behavioral reconditioning in the present, rather than the intensive probing of the past. Through behavioral modification, it is hoped that cures can be achieved in a matter of months, rather than the many years characteristic of traditional psychotherapy.

One major consequence of the Masters and Johnson studies has been the emergence of "sex therapy" as an important and generally recognized field of professional specialization. The practitioners, or "sex therapists," are a diverse group, including individuals with traditional medical training, psychologists, and others with varying backgrounds in personal and family counseling. In general, most sex therapists are strongly influenced by the early Masters and Johnson explanations of sexual dysfunction, and their suggested treatment approaches. There is, however, a significant and growing number of sex therapists who recognize the importance of physical factors in impotence and who are playing an increasingly important role in the overall treatment process.

THE ERA OF MODERN MEDICAL TREATMENT

The restraints of traditional psychotherapy, combined with contemporary sex therapy approaches and a more hospitable environment for human sexuality research, have served to stimulate medical inquiry into treatments involving surgery and drugs. Research in the field, however, dates back a long way.

Research on penile injections can be traced back to 1668 when Regneri de Graaf, by injecting fluid through a syringe, performed a "miracle," raising an erection in the penis of a cadaver. Hormonal treatment dates to at least 1889 when Frenchman Brown-Sequard injected himself with an extract from the testicles of dogs and noted that he was well pleased with the results. Public interest in hormonal therapy was aroused when, in 1918, another researcher working in France, Serge Voronoff, reported that youth could be prolonged by the grafting of cells from monkey testicles into men. For many years, the public was regularly treated to sensationalized stories of the possibility of renewed youth from the use of "monkey glands." It is difficult to trace the use of surgery to correct impotence associated with vascular problems or physical injuries, but by the mid-1930s several successful operations of this nature were reported.

Penile implants date at least to the 1930s. In 1936, N. A. Bogoras, a Russian, used a section of cartilage from a patient's ribs to reconstruct a penis that had been accidentally amputated. The reconstructed penis was reported to have adequate rigidity for intercourse. Implants based on synthetic materials can be traced to the early 1950s. Research on

penile implants accelerated in the 1960s. By the 1970s, standard devices for penile implantation were available on a com-
mercial basis.

In early 1992, a major medical discovery was reported
that, if fully confirmed, reveals one of the final secrets of the
erection and could lead to greatly improved treatment methods. It has been know for sometime that the smooth muscle
cells of the penis play a key role in the initiating and sustaining of the erection. These muscles, which are normally in a
state of tension, must relax for successful erection to take
place. Due to the efforts of Dr. Jacob Rajfer at the University
of California at Los Angeles and his professional colleagues,
it is now thought that the presence of a simple chemical, nitric
oxide, is the key factor in causing the smooth muscles to
relax. As to be discussed in Chapter 7, the injection into the
penis of drugs such as prostaglandin E_1 and papararine is
now being widely used to treat erectile dysfunction. These
drugs are believed to work as a result of their action on the
smooth muscles. The discovery of the nitric oxide factor
could result in safe and effective drugs that promote erectile
function and avoid the obvious inconvenience of injection by
hypodermic syringe into the penis.

Longer term is the promise of the ongoing Genome
Project, a major effort designed to chart the genetic code or
DNA structure that governs the actions of every cell in the
human body. This project could result in gene therapy techniques that reverse the effects of the physical condition that
underlie erectile dysfunction.

Apart from the selected use of the penile implant and
penile injection, there are still no surgical pharmaceutical
solutions to the problem of true psychological impotence.
Research now underway could offer long-range alternatives
to extended psychotherapy or sex therapy. Assuming the
validity of the theory that psychological impotence results

from excessive fear-induced adrenalin production, the use of various substances known as adrenergic blockers that block adrenalin output by the adrenal gland night serve as a solution. Such substances are known to exist, although there is concern as to side effects. It is also potentially dangerous to completely block the adrenalin supply, considering adrenalin's importance in the body's normal response to emergency situations.

After thousands of years, impotence is finally coming out of the closet and practical solutions are now available. The focus has finally shifted from unsupported psychological speculation, blaming the victim for supposed youthful follies, to experimental research and the application of the scientific method. As a result, more has been learned in the past several decades about the causes and effective treatment of impotence than was learned in the past several centuries.

UNDERSTANDING THE MALE SEXUAL MECHANISM

Understanding the causes of impotence and other male sexual problems requires some basic knowledge of the design of the male sexual mechanism and the physical events that should normally take place during sexual intercourse.

Several diagrams in this chapter help explain the mechanical aspects of male sexual behavior. The first, Figure 3-1, shows the various components of the male urinary-genital system, and how they are interconnected. The second, Figure 3-2, shows, in highly simplified form, the all-important vascular or blood supply connections to the interior of the penis. The third, Figure 3-3, reveals the internal structure of the penis and includes the key elements within the penis that make erection possible.

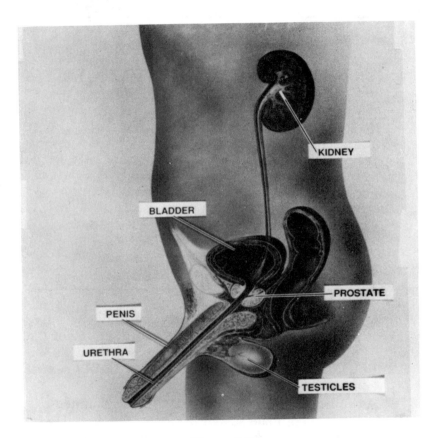

Figure 3-1
Components of the Male Urinary-Genital System
Courtesy of Bard Urological Division, C.R. Bard, Inc.
Illustration by Anthony E. Foote

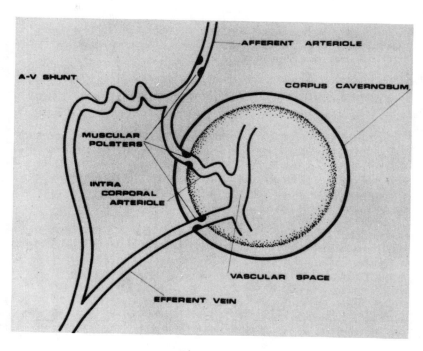

Figure 3-2
Simplified Diagram of the Blood Supply to the Penis

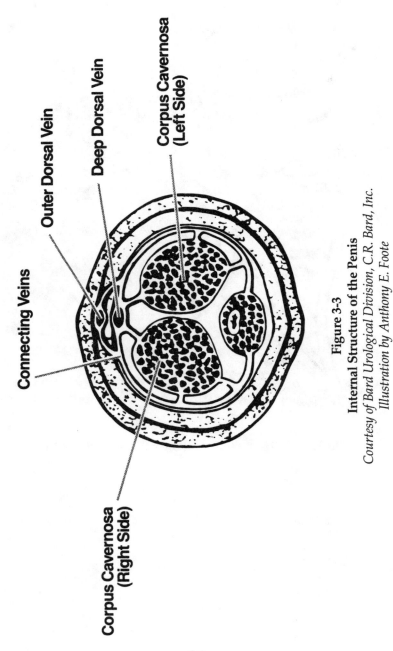

Connecting Veins

Outer Dorsal Vein

Deep Dorsal Vein

Corpus Cavernosa (Left Side)

Corpus Cavernosa (Right Side)

Figure 3-3
Internal Structure of the Penis
Courtesy of Bard Urological Division, C.R. Bard, Inc.
Illustration by Anthony E. Foote

THE MALE URINARY-GENITAL SYSTEM

As its name implies, the male urinary-genital system serves more than one purpose. One of its purposes is to provide the means for the necessary and continuing elimination of liquid wastes from the body in the form of urine. A second purpose is to provide the means for the male contribution to the process of human reproduction. The urinary-genital system also includes facilities that manufacture the vital chemical substances that are critical to growth (especially during puberty) and that contribute to general good health and vigor.

A discussion of the individual components of the male urinary-genital system and their respective functions follows. Also see Figure 3-1 for an illustration of the various components of the male urinary-genital system.

The Penis

The penis is used both for the elimination of urine and for reproduction. In urination, the penis is an important component of the pathway for the flow of urine from the bladder to the outside of the body. The penis is obviously used most of the time for urine elimination. A healthy adult male produces urine at the rate of about a liter (roughly one quart) per day. Over a lifetime, this results in enough liquid to fill an 18-foot-diameter, above-ground backyard swimming pool. In reproduction, the penis serves as the pathway for sperm and spermatic fluid to the outside of the body. Passing ejaculate does not overtax the penis—5 milliliters is the typical total discharge, roughly one teaspoon.

The penis has two other functions with respect to reproduction. First, it serves, when in the erect state, as the means for the deposition of sperm at a point within the female body where chances for successful impregnation are the greatest.

It is also the site where most of the pleasurable physical sensations associated with intercourse and orgasm are concentrated. Such pleasurable sensations, in both men and women, in the absence of the mating cycle as is the case with most other animals, apparently serve to encourage frequent intercourse and hence ensure the propagation of the human species.

A word on penis size. In one scientific investigation, the average nonerect penis length, in a group of fifty men aged 18 to 53, was found to be only 9.3 centimeters (about 3.5 inches). At the same time, the average penis diameter for the group was only 2.9 centimeters (slightly over an inch). According to another report, the length of the erect penis in the average American male is in the 12.7 centimeters (about 5 inches) to 17.8 centimeters (about 7 inches) range. When the penis is erect, an additional 7.6 centimeters (about 3 inches) in length is hidden inside the body.

There are, of course, wide variations from the norm. Rasputin, the "mad monk" of Russia, is reported to have had an erect penis of 33 centimeters (about 13 inches). Napoleon's penis, recently reported to be preserved in a jar at the Columbia University College of Physicians and Surgeons, is said to be only about 5 centimeters (under 2 inches) in length.

There is no evidence that men with smaller penis dimensions are at any tangible disadvantage with respect to sexual performance, or that large penises make a significant impression on most women. History recalls Rasputin for his extraordinary sexual exploits, but Napoleon is also remembered for his accomplishments in this area.

Nevertheless, many men are concerned about penis size, and in some cases, this concern can be valid. The emotional impact is certainly understandable and very real in the case of boys and young men with very small penises who fear ridicule by their often cruel peers in such circumstances as changing clothes in the locker room of a school gym or while showering in a military barracks. In one recent study by psychiatrists, it was found that 70 percent of a group of men who were treated with "talk therapy" for emotional problems associated with tiny penises were able to make a satisfactory adjustment. A significant 30 percent of the men studied were not helped. As to be discussed in Chapter 10, there is now a surgical technique for enhancing the length and girth of the penis available for men who cannot adjust.

The Testicles

The testicles serve as the site for the production of sperm and male sexual hormones, especially testosterone. Some testosterone, however, is also produced in the adrenal glands. An adequate supply of healthy sperm is a critical element in the reproductive process. Sperm, however, is not a factor in the impotence problem. Men with low sperm counts and men who have chosen to have vasectomies are perfectly capable of highly successful sexual intercourse; that is, they are capable of having erections and of successful vaginal penetration. Contrary to popular folklore, the existence of a large family by no means implies extraordinary virility.

Testosterone is a steroid substance that plays a very important role in the processes that take place in the male fetus and in boys during puberty. In the case of the fetus, which in the early stages of development is unisex in nature, testosterone initiates and drives the processes that differentiate potential male babies from female and creates the male sexual organs as seen in the infant at birth. In the absence of testosterone, all babies would be born with female characteristics. In the case of puberty, an inadequate testosterone supply at this important stage of life can result in the failure to develop such normal masculine characteristics as facial and body hair and the typically deep male speaking voice.

In older men, an inadequate supply of testosterone is often associated with loss of libido or sexual desire, and sometimes with the failure to obtain and maintain an erection. Such men may also experience muscular weakness and a general loss of vigor.

The location of the testicles outside the body, in the pouch known as the scrotum, reflects the fact that ideal conditions for sperm production are at temperatures below the normal body temperature of 98.6 degrees Fahrenheit. The old saying to the contrary, a freezing cold day will not result in a loss of the testicles, inhibit sperm production, or impair sperm quality. Remember that collected sperm is often stored frozen and later thawed for artificial insemination. The location of the testicles outside the body cavity does, however, make them more prone to physical injury.

Testicles are formed within the body of the fetus, and sometimes one or even both testicles have not descended into the scrotum at the time of birth. This condition can usually be easily corrected. Incidentally, one testicle normally hangs slightly lower than the other. This configuration reflects a certain lack of symmetry in the internal structure of the human body.

The Prostate and Seminal Vesicles

The prostate is a gland (or, more exactly, a group of glands) enclosed by an outer shell that is unique to men and that is located in a highly confined position under the bladder and in close proximity to the urethra. The prostate serves as the source of about one-half of the whitish fluid known as semen, which carries the sperm. Two glands, known as the seminal vesicles, account for the additional fluid that makes up the semen. These glands are located behind the prostate

The prostate is a frequent source of a variety of problems men may face as they age. The prostate is normally about the size of a golf ball. Very often benign (noncancerous) tumors develop in the prostate. As the gland grows to many times its normal size, it can push down on the urethra with serious urinary problems the end result. Cancerous tumors are another possibility. Prostate cancer is now the leading cause of death from cancer in men. Impotence is often an unavoidable side effect of the treatment of these problems with surgery, radiation, or hormonal drugs. Many men also often experience prostate infections. This sometimes results in premature ejaculation.

Contrary to popular belief, a man can have a fully healthy prostate, but unfortunately still experience erectile difficulty. An erectile problem, however, can be one of the consequences of an unhealthy prostate. Physicians examine the prostate by means of a finger inserted into the rectum, along with other tests. As early detection of prostate problems is important, an annual prostate examination is highly recommended, especially in older men.

The Vas Deferens

Two lengthy tubular structures known as the vas deferens are connected to each testicle and serve as parallel pipelines for the delivery of sperm out of the testicles. The fluid flowing from each vas deferens flows into two intersections analogous to the "T-joints" in plumbing systems. At the T-joints, the fluid originating in the testicles joins and mixes with fluid flowing from each seminal vesicle. The joint stream, plus additional fluid originating in the prostate, ultimately flows through a channel to the urethra.

The surgical severing and tying of each vas deferens constitutes the now-common operative procedure known as a vasectomy. With each vas deferens severed, sperm cannot travel out of the testicles, and the patient, by choice, is rendered infertile. Following a vasectomy, the sperm that continues to be generated in the testicles has no place to go and is harmlessly absorbed in the body. Normal ejaculation of semen, and orgasm, however, continue as before the operation.

A vasectomy in no way affects the production of testosterone or its distribution throughout the body, because the normal route for the movement of testosterone out of the testicles is through the blood system. In short, it is impossible for a vasectomy to physically affect sexual performance. Sometimes men who wrongly equate fertility with potency or have other misconceptions will experience emotional problems following a vasectomy, and in a minor number of cases, there can be adverse consequences with respect to sexual performance.

The Bladder

Because the kidney generates urine on a continuous basis and humans urinate only intermittently, a facility is required for temporary urine storage. This is provided by the saclike structure known as the bladder.

In urination, urine leaving the bladder passes through another plumbing type T-joint and subsequently leaves the body via the penis. During periods of sexual activity, ejaculatory fluid also flows through this T-joint. The passage of urine through the "T", however, is controlled by the sphincter muscle, which acts as a valve to prevent the passage of urine during sexual intercourse as well as the backup of ejaculatory fluid into the bladder. Damage to the sphincter muscle, such as can occur during surgery for prostate problems, can result in the flow of ejaculatory fluid into the bladder or incontinence (loss of control over urine flow).

THE BLOOD SUPPLY TO THE PENIS

The importance of the blood supply to the penis cannot be overemphasized. Figure 3-2 shows a simplified diagram of the blood supply to the penis. The blood supply to any part of the body, of course, is critical in view of the role of the blood in the supply of nutrients and oxygen to the tissues, the removal of waste products, and the transport of immunological agents, hormones, and other essential chemical entities. In the case of the penis, the blood supply serves a unique function. As will be discussed in detail shortly, blood acts as a hydraulic fluid that makes penile erection possible.

Blood is pumped to the penis by the heart through the same arterial system that supplies the legs and other locations in the lower body. As the blood moves downstream, it branches out into the large penile artery. This artery then splits within the penis into three major paired arterial systems: the deep artery system, the dorsal artery system and the bulbosa artery system. Each of these systems in turn branches into innumerable channels, which supply various portions of the penis.

The dorsal arteries and associated dorsal veins are familiar to most men, since they can be faintly seen under the skin of the penis. The deep arteries, however, are the most important in erection, because they supply blood to the tissues known as the corpus cavernosum, the site of the erectile process.

While arteries carry blood upstream into the penis, veins carry blood downstream from the penis through what is known as the venous blood system and back to the heart. The extensive network of veins within the corpus cavernosum is also believed to play a key role in the erection process.

THE NERVE SUPPLY TO THE PENIS

Autonomic and somatic nerve circuits interconnect the penis with nerve centers in the brain and key nerve bundles in the spinal column. The functioning of the autonomic section of the nervous system is unconscious in nature and largely beyond one's voluntary control. In addition to controlling some of the actions of the penis, it controls such important activities as the function of the digestive system, blood vessel dilation, maintenance of body temperature, blood pressure, and heart beat. The functioning of the somatic nervous system is conscious in nature. It serves to control such conscious activities as reading the words on this page. Electrical impulses provide the means for the transmission of information through both the autonomic and somatic nerve circuits. It is interesting to note in this connection that ejaculation has been experimentally achieved by stimulation from an external electrical source.

The autonomic and somatic nervous systems both play a role in the erection process. The autonomic system is divided into two subsystems, the parasympathetic and the sympathetic. Of the two, the former is the one involved in the unconscious processes associated with initiating an erection, not only during periods of sexual activity, but also during sleep, or when the penis is unconsciously physically stimulated. The somatic nervous system serves as the electrical pathway for the transmission of conscious images, including erotic images that serve to trigger the chemical and physical processes that take place in erection and the pleasurable sensations associated with sexual activities. The somatic system also helps your penis return to a flaccid state after sexual activities have been concluded.

THE MECHANICS OF ERECTION

Erection and ejaculation should not be confused. Erection is necessary to provide the penis with sufficient rigidity to permit the penetration of the female vagina. Ejaculation, however can be achieved by masturbation in the absence of an erection, although this implies a loss of much of the pleasure associated with sexual relations and presents an obvious, but not unsurmountable, problem with respect to having children.

In humans, erection is achieved by a hydraulic mechanism. Hydraulic systems are based on the inherent difficulty of compressing any kind of liquid. As a result, when a force is applied to a liquid confined within a limited area, a buildup of pressure occurs, and the liquid will press against its physical boundaries.

The brake systems found in modern automobiles are hydraulic in nature. When the driver presses the brake pedal, the considerable pressure buildup activates the braking process. Hydraulic brake systems normally work very well and, for this reason, were adopted many years ago for use in automobiles in preference to simple mechanical braking systems. As every driver knows, hydraulic brakes sometime fail, particularly when leaks occur in the vicinity of the seals. With the penis, leakage of hydraulic fluid, in this case, blood, is one of the possible causes of loss of an erection.

Incidentally, some types of whales do not employ the hydraulic approach for the formidable task of coitus on the high seas. Instead, such whales are equipped with a penile bone. Many men are now employing something very similar, in the form of a penile implant.

To understand how hydraulic forces make an erection possible, it is useful to examine Figure 3-3, the diagram showing the internal structure of the penis. As can be seen from the diagram, "corpus cavernosum" (plural, "corpora cavernosa") tissue, shaped into two long cylinders, parallels the shaft of the penis and the urethral channel over most of their respective lengths. Surrounding, and protecting the corpora cavernosa is a strong fibrous tissue layer known as the tunica albuginea. When conditions call for an erection, the tissues of the corpora cavernosa absorb large quantities of the hydraulic fluid (blood), resulting in the expansion of penis length, diameter, and needed rigidity.

Within the corpus cavernosum are thousands of expandable saclike structures, known as sinuses, each capable of storing very large quantities of blood. The sinuses are surrounded by "smooth" muscle tissue. Smooth muscles are one of the three types of muscles found in the body. The other two are the skeletal muscles, a familiar example being the bicep muscles that control motion in our forearms, and the cardiac muscles that make up the tissue of our hearts. In addition to the functioning of the penis, smooth muscles are involved in such automatic processes as the digestion of food, the elimination of body wastes, and the regulation of blood flow. In contrast to the situation that takes place when we consciously flex our biceps, we normally are unaware and have no conscious control over the functioning of our smooth muscles. The smooth muscles, however, play a key role in erection, contributing both to the flow of blood into the sinuses and the retention of blood within the sinuses during the period the erection is sustained.

Exactly how the sinuses fill with blood during an erection is still subject to some uncertainty, although research now underway may soon provide a full explanation. From the standpoint of hydraulics, filling the sinuses with blood logically involves the continuous pumping of upstream or arterial blood into the sinus cavities and some form of valving action to restrict the downstream movement of blood from the cavities into the veins of the venous blood system. Part of the explanation is that as the sinuses fill with blood, the engorged muscular tissue confined within the rigid envelope of the tunica albuginea cannot expand outward and instead presses internally against the veins that normally transport blood away from the penis. This restricts all but a necessary trickle of the downstream flow. This does not account, however, for how the buildup of blood in the sinuses occurs in the first place.

One possible way to increase the flow of blood into the sinuses would be to substantially increase the pumping rate of the heart. The variations in heartbeat that occur during periods of sexual activity are not sufficient in themselves to account for buildup of blood in the sinuses. A better explanation is that the flow of blood into the sinuses is enhanced due to actions that take place in the smooth muscle tissues. An important characteristic of smooth muscles is that they are most of the time under tension and in a contracted state. While thus contracted, the smooth muscles, within the corpus cavernosum, normally constrict the arteries, that is, reduce the inside diameter of the arteries, that carry blood into the penis. When an erection occurs, however, the smooth muscles relax. This, in turn, allows the arteries to expand and greatly increase the flow of blood into sinuses within the penis.

The erection has been defined as a multifaceted process initiated by events with the nervous system and then maintained by a complex interplay between the vascular system and the nervous system. The most likely sequence of events is that the erection first gets underway when appropriate messages are sent to the nerve centers in the penis that directly control the smooth muscles of the corpus cavernosum. This, in turn, serves to dilate (increase the inside diameter) of the arteries entering the corpus cavernosum, resulting in increased blood flow. Then, as the erection process gains momentum, the valving action in the exiting veins come into play. It is also reasonable to conclude that feedback relationships probably exist between the indicated upstream and downstream mechanisms. When all goes well, there is a major increase in the internal blood pressure of the corpus cavernosum, to well above normal body reading. The rise indicates that both the filling and valving mechanisms are operating properly.

As mentioned in Chapter 2, a very important area of current research is the processes involved in the relaxation of the smooth muscles of the penis. For relaxation to take place, chemical substances that make the smooth muscles relax must be made available within the corpus cavernosum. Nitric oxide is receiving attention as the most likely chemical agent, although other chemicals may be involved, or perhaps a combination of chemicals. Nitric oxide was first investigated in connection with treating cardiovascular disease. The substance, which acts as a neurotransmitter, has been found to be a factor in relaxing the smooth muscles controlling the flow of blood through the major arteries of the body. When these smooth muscles relax, the arteries dilate, resulting in a lowering of blood pressure. Nitric oxide is now also believed to play an important role in the operation of the immune system, including the defense of the body against cancer.

Nitric oxide, a very simple chemical, is best known to the public as a major, and very undesirable, constituent of smog and acid rain. The removal of nitric oxide from automobile exhaust emissions is one of the principal functions of the catalytic devices that are now installed in all automobiles. It is ironic that this toxic substance may prove to be an invaluable agent in the treatment not only of impotence, but also many other physical disorders.

An important area of current investigation is exactly how nitric oxide is generated within the corpus cavernosum. There is now reason to believe that messages sent from the brain to nerve centers within the smooth muscles of the penis result in the generation and release of nitric oxide. The living cells of the body, including those of the nervous system, are proteins in nature. Proteins, in turn, are formed from simpler substances known as amino acids, chemicals whose composition includes nitrogen and oxygen. Interest now centers on the essential amino acid, l-arginine. There are grounds to suspect that the messages sent to the penis result in the breakdown of l-arginine yielding the all-important nitric oxide.

Finally, it is important to consider the processes that take place within the brain and nervous system that result in appropriate messages to the penis. The erection is essentially a reflex action that cannot be consciously willed. Sometimes an erection is triggered by psychological factors when the center in the brain associated with the functions of the somatic nervous system is activated by intimate contact with a sexual partner or by merely viewing or even imagining erotic images. An erection may also be triggered via the parasympathetic nervous system when nerve centers located in the spinal cord are stimulated by the physical stroking of the penis. Typically, both processes take place simultaneously. It is also typical, as men age, for the erection to become more dependent upon direct physical stimulation of the penis, a factor that should be recognized during sexual relations.

Erections are, of course, expected to take place during periods of sexual activities with a partner or during masturbation. In healthy men, erections also normally occur about three to six times per night, while asleep and during dream periods. Such nocturnal erections may last for up to 30 minutes and are often observed by men when awakening. Studies have shown that nocturnal erections can often occur during dreams that have no erotic content. This seems to indicate that nocturnal erections are largely controlled by the autonomic nervous system.

The reasons for nocturnal erections are not fully known, but such erections may represent the way the body checks on whether the erectile mechanism is working properly, in much the same manner that aerospace engineers repeatedly check key mechanical systems prior to launching a complicated space vehicle.

THE MECHANICS OF EJACULATION

Ejaculation occurs as a result of vigorous contractions of muscles in the vicinity of the urethra, the prostate, and in the general pelvic area. The pumping action provided by the contractions is similar to what occurs at the beach when you quickly squeeze the surface of the water with a cupped hand and observe the resulting upright spurt.

Ejaculation, of course, has as its primary purpose the delivery of seminal fluid essential for human reproduction. It also serves to relieve the prostate of excess seminal fluid. A portion of the total volume of seminal fluid is continuously produced within the prostate. In the absence of periodic ejaculation, the prostate can become often painfully "congested," due to a buildup of excess fluid. This often occurs in sexually abstinent men. In the absence of sexual relations or nocturnal emissions, the buildup can be relieved by masturbation or possibly prostate massage by a urologist.

The contractions causing the expulsion of seminal fluid are reflexes that are neurological in nature and normally extend to the area of the anus. The complete interrelation of the nerve connections in this general area serves as the basis for several tests discussed in Chapter 5, which may be easily performed in the privacy of the home.

Prior to the moment of ejaculation, a quantity of semen collects in the urethra. The channel connecting the urethra to the bladder is normally closed by the sphincter muscle, while the pathways upstream through the vas deferens are too small to permit reverse fluid flow. Under these circumstances, the muscular contractions can only result in the movement of fluid downstream, through the urethra, and out the tip of the penis.

There is some evidence that chemical substances of an amine nature known as prostaglandins play a role in ejaculation. A large number of different prostaglandins have been detected in human semen. These substances, which are known to be smooth muscle stimulants, could be a factor in the contractions of the prostate and seminal vesicles that occur during ejaculation. Research in this area may result in better methods for dealing with the problem of ejaculatory failure that occurs in some men.

The pleasurable sensations that take place during ejaculation are not dependent upon the presence of the semen. Surgical removal of the prostate results in the absence of the ejaculatory fluid. It is, nevertheless, still possible to experience most of the physical sensations of ejaculation, provided there has been minimal damage to critical nerve connections.

The pleasurable sensations that occur at the moment of ejaculation are, of course, those associated with male orgasm. In the Masters and Johnson studies of the 1960s, a male sexual response cycle was defined in which the events that take place during sexual activities are divided into successive "excitement", "plateau," "orgasm," and "resolution" stages. In orgasm, two substages have been identified: a period of ejaculatory inevitability and a period of actual ejaculation. The short period of ejaculatory inevitability is believed to take place at the time when substantial quantities of semen collect in the urethra. The awareness that ejaculation is imminent and irreversible is a very familiar feeling to most men.

During the resolution stage that follows ejaculation, the erection is normally quickly lost. In the shutdown process, nerve impulses direct the relaxation of the muscles of the corpus cavernosum. This results, in turn, in the decreased flow of upstream arterial blood, the collapse of the sinus cavities, and the rapid downstream flow of the blood that had been temporarily stored within the penis.

THINGS THAT CAN GO WRONG

The male urinary-genital system normally works remarkably well, considering its overall complexity and restricted geometry. However, one inherent design flaw is the combination of the urinary and genital functions. As any engineer can attest, the tying together of functional systems in any complicated device, such as an automobile, means that a failure in one system will, more than likely, result in trouble in all the other interrelated systems, and possibly total incapacitation. The female body, incidentally, is more logically designed, in that there is a complete separation of the equipment used for urination and that used for reproduction.

The tight geometry of the male urinary-genital system results in problems similar to those faced by the automobile mechanic working under the crowded hood of a modern motor vehicle. In this respect, men do have an advantage over women—in the female body there is even less space to work in when something goes wrong.

Impotence has always been the most common problem of the male urinary-genital system with respect to successful sexual performance. The causes of impotence are discussed in the next chapter. There are other problems that men experience, such as premature ejaculation, that can often be just as troubling. These problems, which are discussed in Chapter 5, may have a serious impact on health and well-being. Examples include infections of the prostate and urethra; tumors of the prostate, testicles, and bladder; kidney stones; and the general problem of male infertility. While a general discussion of these problems is beyond the scope of this book, some of these problems can contribute to dysfunction and are relevant in this sense.

Any patient diagnosed as having one of the foregoing problems would be well advised to bear in mind the possibility of a connection between his medical condition and impotence, and certainly should discuss this with his doctor if he has any of the symptoms of impotence.

CHAPTER 4

WHAT
CAUSES
IMPOTENCE

Given the way erection takes place, it is logical to conclude that impotence is essentially a problem caused by one or more negative factors impacting in some way on the vascular system transporting blood through the penis or the nerve connections involved in sending messages calling for erections to the penis. In some cases, a single factor affecting either the blood supply or the nerve connections may underlie the problem. Other cases may be more complicated, with multiple factors at work. The possibility of impotence of a psychological nature is by no means precluded. When psychological factors are at work, they can be manifested only via chemical agents transported through the bloodstream or electrical impulses transmitted via the nervous system.

The problems that are known to cause impotence under some circumstances may be logically grouped as follows:

◆ Problems that mainly affect the flow of blood into the penis and the ability of the penis to retain sufficient blood to maintain an erection

◆ Problems that mainly affect that portion of the nervous system that serves the penis

◆ Other problems that significantly affect both the vascular and nervous systems or those in which the mechanism is currently not fully understood

BLOOD FLOW AND RETENTION PROBLEMS

Blood flow, or "vasculogenic," problems that may adversely affect erection can occur on either the upstream (arterial) side of the penis or on the downstream (venous) side. On the upstream side, it is reasonable to suspect anything that diminishes the flow of arterial blood to the penis as a possible cause of impotence. These include the following:

◆ Narrowing and hardening of arteries

◆ Blockage of arteries

◆ Thickening of the blood

On the downstream side, abnormal leakage of blood out of the sinus cavities can result in impotence. A number of factors may account for such leakage.

Narrowing and Hardening of Arteries

In the typical male, the average inside diameter of each of the deep penile arteries that supply blood to the corpus cavernosum is in the 1.5- to 3.0-millimeter (about 0.06- to 0.12-inch) range. At the lower end of the range, the diameter is smaller than the head of a pin. Because these tight dimensions provide very little excess flow capacity, any further reduction in size is capable of causing problems. Some men are also just born with very narrow arteries, and unfortunately may have a potential problem built into their systems.

Arteriosclerosis, a leading cause of death in older men and women, is also a major factor underlying male impotence. In the very common form of arteriosclerosis popularly known as hardening of the arteries, the interior arterial walls throughout the body gradually become lined with deposits of fatty substances over a period of time. This buildup of deposits results in both a constriction of the lumen, or inside arterial channel, and a decrease in arterial elasticity. Under these circumstances, there is a reduction in the normal flow of blood through the flaccid or nonerect penis. Even worse, the penile arteries will not sufficiently dilate to permit increased blood flow when the signal arrives through the nervous system calling for an erection. When these problems occur, tests in the urologist's office will usually reveal penile blood pressure readings at well below adequate levels.

The problem is somewhat analogous to what you may encounter in the plumbing of an old house, especially in an area supplied with highly mineralized water. Should you turn on a faucet and to your frustration only get a trickle, you will probably complain about the lack of pressure and call for a plumber. After completing the job, the plumber will more than likely show you an old section of pipe and point out how the inside walls are almost entirely coated with a white and very hard deposit of minerals. Unfortunately, replacing old arteries takes more of an effort than does replacing old pipe.

A common symptom indicating some degree of arteriosclerosis is pain in the legs after vigorously walking for some distance. This symptom suggests the possibility of peripheral vascular disease (PVD), a disorder resulting from inadequate arterial blood flow to the legs. It is not surprising that 40 to 80 percent of all men with PVD also suffer from erectile dysfunction.

The use of tobacco products, especially cigarettes, has been clearly linked to both impotence and the increased statistical risk of heart disease. Substances in tobacco smoke have been found to cause significant blood vessel constriction. On occasion, some impotence patients have even experienced greatly improved erectile function following the cessation of smoking. The male smoker, therefore, faces the increased long-range risk of becoming impotent, due to the consequences of heart disease, and a more immediate risk from the direct effects of tobacco.

Radiation therapy in the vicinity of the penis can result in impotence. Radiation therapy is often called for in cases of cancer of the prostate or bladder. Scarring of tissue in all forms of radiation therapy is very common. When the blood vessels of the penis are scarred, they lose the elasticity needed for proper penile blood flow during erections. Nerve damage may also occur.

Radiation therapy for prostate cancer can be either of the external beam radiotherapy or seed implantation type. In the former, in which the prostate is bombarded by a focused beam of X rays from an external machine, impotence can be the result in 20 to 40 percent of all patients treated. In the latter, in which tiny capsules of radioactive substances are surgically implanted into the prostate, impotence can be the result in up to 10 percent of all patients treated. The good news is that recent clinical trials of a new form of seed implantation radiation therapy that employs palladium 103, along with Iodine 125, as the radioactive substances, has been shown to result in a much lower occurrence of impotence.

Blockage of Arteries

Impotence can result from any significant blockage at a critical point in the major arteries serving the penis. Blockages can result from operative procedures, physical injury, and the aging process alone. Whenever surgery is performed on the major blood vessels of the body, there is always some danger of a small fatty deposit, known as an embolus, breaking loose, flowing downstream, and lodging at some point, thus creating a blockage.

Blockages can also be caused by certain types of physical injuries to the pelvic region that result in obstruction of one or more of the major arteries. With age, blockages can occur in the major blood vessels leading to the legs. Such blockages can make walking difficult and sometimes painful. Since the arteries to the penis split off from the arteries leading to the legs, it is very common for men experiencing such blockages to simultaneously experience problems with erections.

Thickening of the Blood

Decreased flow of blood to the penis may occur in conditions that result in a thickening or loss of fluidity of the blood. Blood can take on a sludgelike character in individuals suffering from sickle-cell anemia, a genetic disease largely experienced by persons of African and Mediterranean ancestry. Chemotherapy, used in the treatment of certain kinds of cancer, can also result in a similar effect on blood.

This condition, however, may reverse following the conclusion of the chemotherapy program.

Abnormal Leakage of Blood

Men subject to leakage of venous blood from the sinus cavities experience semirigid erections or, more commonly, reasonably firm erections that are quickly lost, typically within a period of about 2 minutes. A condition known as an arterial venous malformation, in which there is a defective connection between the arteries and the veins, may be at the root of the problem. Defective valving action on the venous side, or inadequate filling of the sinus cavities, can also be a factor. When this is the case, the underlying cause may be that the tissues inside the corpora cavernosa have lost their elasticity and ability to relax adequately. When this is the case the tissues do not properly expand and thus fail to exert sufficient pressure to restrict flow through the veins carrying blood away from the penis.

The loss of function of the tissues inside the penis is now believed to be the consequence of much the same underlying factors as discussed earlier in connection with arterial constriction and blockage problems, including arteriosclerosis and use of tobacco. It is now also generally thought that such leakage abnormalities account for the largest share of vasculogenic disorders associated with erectile failure.

PROBLEMS IN THE NERVOUS SYSTEM

The following problems primarily affecting the nervous system have been identified as possible causes of impotence:

◆ Alcohol abuse
◆ Illegal substance abuse

◆ Use of certain prescription and nonprescription drugs

◆ Surgery and physical injury

◆ Neurological disorders

◆ Psychological factors

Chapter 5 describes some simple tests that you can perform yourself to determine whether you have suffered nerve damage.

Alcohol Abuse

The abuse of alcohol can play a very significant role in impotence. Moderate alcohol consumption has been said to have an aphrodisiac effect. In moderation, the effect can be an increase in libido and the reduction of social and sexual inhibitions. With heavier drinking, the central nervous system is subject to depression, and the drinker typically experiences some loss of control over mental and physical faculties. Even younger men in excellent health and with no history of sexual dysfunction can experience episodes of temporary impotence when drunk. Such situations only reconfirm the sad truth of Shakespeare's words, that alcohol "provokes the desire, but takes away the performance" (*Macbeth*, Act II, Scene 3).

Moderate social drinking does not seem to represent a major contributory factor to chronic persistent impotence. At some point, however, a significant portion of the population crosses the line between moderate social drinking and the alcohol dependency syndrome better known as alcoholism. The usual symptoms of alcoholism are early morning drinking, a consistent heavy daily intake, and withdrawal symptoms during periods of abstinence. Perhaps as many as 5 percent of the U.S. male population typically become alcoholics, probably as a consequence of their inherent metabolic profiles programmed into their genes.

Alcoholism in both men and women frequently results in serious impairment of the peripheral nervous system. Damage is cumulative and in males extends to the nerves controlling the bulbocavernosus reflex in the penis. The result can be irreversible damage that will continue into the future despite regained sobriety.

Alcoholism also takes its toll as a result of its typical effect on the body's hormonal balances. High estrogen and low testosterone levels are often detected in male alcoholics. The liver, an organ often seriously damaged by alcohol abuse, can be an important factor in this occurrence. As the normal function of the liver is impaired, the level of the female hormone, estrogen, rises in the bloodstream. At the same time, testosterone levels drop, due to the increased breakdown of the male hormone by the liver. Alcohol also inhibits the production of testosterone in the testicles. As a result, testosterone levels may be reduced even in the absence of severe liver damage.

The hormonal abnormalities that are often seen in male alcoholics can clearly have an impact on sexual characteristics and function. For example, noticeable breast and nipple enlargement often takes place in chronic alcohol abusers.

The impotent alcoholic's difficulties are often compounded by heavy smoking, use of various illegal substances, poor diet, and overeating. The combination frequently has synergistic consequences that work together to exacerbate the problem. Overeating, leading to obesity, is often associated with heart disease and high blood pressure. The medications used to treat these problems often result in impotence. Finally, the usual pattern of vitamin deficiency and emotional stress in male alcoholics may also add to the impotence problem.

This combination of problems that often exists for the male alcoholic is illustrated by the profile of George, age 60, who was treated for impotence.

George, a construction worker, reported that it is very common for workers in the building trades to drink heavily on the job. In fact, many employers routinely provide large quantities of beer, in the belief that this stimulates production. George has had previous surgery for prostate cancer and had been taking prescription drugs linked to impotence to treat high blood pressure and ulcers. A penile implant proved the only solution for his impotence.

Illegal Substance Abuse

All the common mind-altering substances usually bought and consumed on an illegal basis (street drugs) are suspect when it comes to impotence. The level of use at which problems will develop with these substances is even less clear than with alcohol, given the obvious impediments to scientific research in this area.

Marijuana (cannabis), in the past the most widely used illegal substance, is relatively benign with respect to impotence and, in general, appears to represent less of a problem than alcohol. While marijuana is known to lower a man's sperm count, there is no demonstrated connection between a low sperm count and erectile dysfunction. Use of marijuana and associated substances, such as hashish, does appear to lower testosterone levels slightly and thus could have an effect on sexual desire (libido). Fortunately, the effect on testosterone is usually short term and reversible. It is worth noting, however, that there are some reports in the medical literature linking erectile dysfunction to long-term marijuana use. There are also some reports that prolonged use of marijuana can affect the pituitary gland and result in an increased level of production in the bloodstream. Prolactin is the key hormone responsible for the production of breast milk in women. This would suggest, although not fully proven, that a mechanism exists by which the use of marijuana could result in the loss of some degree of male sexual function.

The use of cocaine, known in its concentrated form as crack, has grown significantly in recent years as the illegal drug industry has shifted its operations away from marijuana to a product that offers a much greater financial return for the same degree of risk. Cocaine is potentially far more serious with respect to impotence and other health problems. Male cocaine users sometimes report increased libido the first few times the drug is consumed. Long-term habitual users, however, very often report partial or complete loss of erection. The drug is known to have an adverse effect on the central and peripheral nervous systems. Amphetamines, such as speed, have similar effects on the central and peripheral nervous systems, and are also implicated in impotence. Little is known regarding the effect of lysergic acid (LSD) on erectile function, although the fact that the drug does have a strong effect on the nervous system suggests that there could be a possible impact.

Opium derivatives, such as heroin, are currently reported to be regaining their past popularity. Such drugs are thought to act as aphrodisiacs in very small doses. Consumption of larger quantities and habitual use can result in decreased libido and nervous system damage contributing to impotence. Similar problems may result from methadone, a synthetic heroin substitute that is often legally provided to narcotics abusers in treatment programs.

Use of Certain Prescription and Nonprescription Drugs

Impotence is a possible side effect of a broad spectrum of drugs commonly used in the treatment of various medical problems. Most of the time such drugs are available only on a prescription basis; however, problems can exist with some drugs sold on an over-the-counter basis. A listing of products that have been linked in various reports to impotence is given in Appendix A. If you are taking any of the prescribed products in Appendix A and are experiencing erectile difficulties, it is important that you first consult with your physician and obtain approval before discontinuing use. Failure to do so in some cases could have very serious consequences. It is also important to recognize that people react differently to drugs and that a drug that might cause erectile failure in one man may have no adverse effect on another.

Problems are most common in the case of cardiovascular preparations, which include drugs used in the treatment of high blood pressure and various heart and vascular system problems. Frequently prescribed brand-name drugs in which impotence problems have been encountered include Aldomet, Serpasil, Inderal, and Lopressor. Exactly how the various cardiovascular preparations act to cause impotence is still not fully understood, and the exact mechanism may also vary from drug to drug. It has been suggested that many drugs of this type inhibit the normal function of the neurotransmitters that control the dilation of the critical blood vessels of the corpus cavernosum. These drugs have in many cases been associated with other undesirable side effects, including lethargy, insomnia, and problems in concentration. As a consequence, there is an ongoing shift to drugs of the calcium channel blocker and ACE inhibitor type, which typically have fewer side effects.

Many drugs used for the control of emotional states have been linked to impotence. These include tranquilizers and antianxiety preparations ("downers") and antidepressants ("uppers"). In the former category are such brand-name products as Valium, Librium, Equanil, and Thorazine. The latter category includes such brand-name drugs as Elavil and Tofranil. It is worth noting that depression is a frequent side effect of drugs used to treat high blood pressure. Such circumstances may present a patient with a double impotence risk.

A partial list of the types of drugs that have also been linked to impotence includes barbiturates, sedatives, sleeping pills, and antihistamines. These drugs are believed to alter, in some manner, the proper functioning of the central nervous system. The widely prescribed brand-name drug Tagamet (cimetidine) used in the treatment of ulcers has been linked to impotence. Other side effects of this drug may include decreased libido and lethargy. The use of Tagamet, similar to that of marijuana, can result in an increased level of the hormone production. Some other drugs that have been linked to possible increased levels of production include Haldol (haloperidol), Janimine (imipramine), Tofranil (imipramine), and Aldomet (methylodopa).

Estrogen therapy is still sometimes employed in the treatment of benign prostate hyperplasia (BPH) and cancer of the prostate, although improved drugs have made their appearance in recent years. Typical effects of the use of the female hormone are reduced libido and impotence. Estrogen has often been employed in quack cures for male baldness. Most of these cures have fortunately involved the use of the hormone in salves and lotions applied to the skin on a topical basis. As such, they have probably not contributed to impotence. They have also not contributed to the desired growth of hair.

Erectile dysfunction is a possible consequence of the use of flutamine, a drug sold under the brand name Eulexin for the treatment of both benign and malignant prostate tumors. Proscar, the brand name of a drug that has received considerable recent attention as a treatment for benign prostate tumors, is reported to result in reversible impotence in about 3.5 percent of all users. Impotence is also a possible consequence of the use of leuprolide, a drug sold under the brand name Lupron for the treatment of prostate cancer.

Cigarette smoking is reported to increase the probability of impotence in men taking prescription drugs. According to the recent Massachusetts Male Aging Study, smoking cigarettes increased the age-adjusted probability of complete impotence in men taking cardiac drugs from 14 to 41 percent, antihypertensive medication from 7.5 to 21 percent, and vasodilators from 21 to 52 percent.

Surgery, Radiation Therapy, and Physical Injury

Impotence can result from nerve damage during various types of surgery. This includes surgery for benign enlargement of the prostate; cancer of the prostate, bladder, rectum, and anus; aortic aneurysm resection; and aortal femoral bypass. Surgery in the prostate region can also result in blood supply problems that may result in impotence. In the case of men with prostate cancer who have experienced a radical prostatectomy (complete surgical removal of the prostate), impotence occurs in up to 70 percent of all cases. New surgical techniques have been developed in recent years that are intended to minimize the damage to vital nerve connections during prostate and related surgery for cancer of the bladder and rectum. The jury of medical opinion is still out on the degree of effectiveness of such procedures. The results in some patients have been encouraging, although the techniques, in general, would appear to require further refinement.

As previously indicated, radiation therapy in the vicinity of the penis can result in impotence due to damage of a vascular nature. Such therapy can also result in nerve damage contributing to erectile failure. As discussed, new techniques based on seed implantation offer hope in this area.

Surgical removal of the testicles (orchiectomy) is sometimes necessitated in cases of cancer of the prostate and in connection with testicular cancer, which is not as common. Impotence is frequently experienced after such surgery. Some men, however, are still able to obtain erections and experience satisfactory intercourse despite having an orchiectomy. This was sometime found to be true in the case of castrated men employed as eunuchs in the harems of China and the Ottoman Empire.

Impotence can also be caused by nerve damage resulting from accidental damage or trauma. As previously noted, severe injuries to the pelvic region may result in impotence, due to obstructions in the arterial blood vessels supplying the penis. Such injuries may often result in serious nerve damage. Trouble can be expected in approximately one-third of the cases of male pelvic damage.

Spinal cord injuries often result in impotence. The extent of erectile failure, as well as paralysis throughout the body and other physical problems, depends on the location and severity of the damage. The situation is complicated, but, in general, the less the spinal cord has been severed and the lower down the injury occurs, the better the overall prognosis. When the cord has been only partially severed, erections are still often possible, although in many instances, they are of short duration. Injuries at the higher end of the column typically prevent the transmission of erotic thoughts from the brain to the penis to stimulate erections. Such individuals, however, may still have erections of the reflex type with appropriate mechanical stimulation. In treating individuals with spinal cord injuries, efforts to restore sexual function are very important to the patient's overall emotional condition. Research is underway that offers the promise of electrically stimulated ejaculation when such patients want to father children.

Impotence can result, on occasion, from direct physical injury to the penis, either by nerve or blood vessel damage.

Unless the damage has been too severe, function usually returns in time. At times, surgery will be necessitated. An unusual case was that of Tony, age 38, who injured his penis by falling on a tree stump while deer hunting. The injury resulted in Peyronie's disease, a condition characterized by a seriously bent penis. A surgical procedure was successful in restoring the normal shape of the penis, but a penile implant was eventually required to restore proper sexual function.

Neurological Disorders

Various neurological problems can result in impotence. These include both benign and malignant tumors of the brain and spinal cord. Multiple sclerosis (MS), a progressive disease that attacks the brain and spinal cord, causes great weakness and degeneration of the peripheral regions of the body. Impotence, due to damage to the nerve circuits serving the penis, also results in about 25 percent of all MS cases. Impotence problems of a neurological nature also may appear in men subject to epilepsy and Parkinson's disease.

PROBLEMS OF BOTH THE BLOOD SUPPLY AND THE NERVOUS SYSTEM

Diabetes

Blood supply and nervous system problems resulting in impotence often occur when a man has diabetes mellitus. Diabetes, when untreated, is a potentially life-threatening disease in both men and women. In diabetes, failure of the pancreas to secrete sufficient quantities of the vital substance insulin results in the inability of the body to metabolize carbohydrates properly in the form of sugars and starches. *About one-half of all men in whom diabetes has been detected will typically develop impotence over a ten-year period following the onset of the disease.* Control of diabetes is extremely important through diet and regular visits to your physician.

Diabetes may first occur in childhood or in later life. Juvenile diabetes is generally more serious than adult diabetes, although it can be more rapidly detected and treated. Adult diabetes often develops over a period of time and has less obvious symptoms. Often, the first symptom of adult diabetes in men is impotence. For this reason, any man experiencing impotence is well advised to have appropriate urinalysis and blood tests performed to check on the possibility of diabetes. As there is evidence that diabetes involves genetic factors, men with a family history of the disease who experience impotence problems should be especially cautious. Penile fibrosis, a condition in which scar tissue forms within the penis, is also much more common in the diabetic patient.

Vascular disease is believed to represent the most immediate factor causing impotence in diabetic men. Arteriosclerosis, associated with diabetes, results in problems in both the large and small blood vessels of the body, including lesions of the deep penile arteries. The disease, after a period of time, also usually results in serious damage to both the somatic and autonomic nervous systems. Often, matters are complicated in adult male diabetics by obesity and alcoholism. The high blood glucose levels experienced by men with improperly controlled diabetes can also be a significant factor. Such levels result in general fatigue, malaise, and depression, all of which contribute to psychological impotence and diminished libido.

Kidney Disease and Hyperlactinemia

In chronic kidney disease, kidney failure often results in abnormal hormone levels that may affect erection. The problems of such patients are often complicated by high blood pressure and the side effects of medications for treating hypertension. There may also be direct damage to nerve circuits leading to the penis.

Kidney failure is life threatening and may require hemodialysis, in which patients must report frequently to treatment centers where they undergo blood filtration using an external artificial kidney. Such treatment is highly stressful and could contribute to psychological impotence in male patients. There is also reason to suspect that the process may result in chemical changes in the mineral content of the bloodstream that contribute to impotence.

Hyperlactinemia is a condition characterized by excess levels of the hormone prolactin, which is secreted by the pituitary gland, a small gland at the base of the skull. As previously mentioned, excess levels of prolactin may be associated with smoking marijuana and the taking of certain prescription drugs such as Tagamet (cimetidine). The most likely cause of hyperlactinemia, however, is a pituitary adenoma (tumor). The drug bromoscriptine is often used to treat such tumors.

Psychological Factors

Psychological factors, acting primarily through the nervous system, may result in impotence, although little is conclusively known about the exact mechanism through which this occurs. Psychological problems such as anxiety, deep depression, guilt, and relationship conflicts are believed to dampen erotic sensations and reduce sensory awareness. As episodes of impotence occur with increasing frequency, the result can be a growing fear of being able to perform in a sexually adequate manner, which, in turn, contributes to erectile difficulties.

The theory, as noted in Chapter 2, that psychological impotence operates through an "adrenalin reflex" may apply best to episodes of temporary impotence, especially in younger men. A sudden rush of adrenalin, of course, occurs in highly fearful situations. Ribald stories about the narrow escape of a young lover, when surprised by an irate husband in *flagrante delicto* are common to all cultures. The typical story often contains the comic image of the young man leaping from the wife's second-story bedchamber, while simultaneously attempting to pull on a pair of pants (or perhaps adjust a toga). Implicit in such stories is the almost instantaneous loss of erection that occurs under such circumstances.

Fearful situations of this type are uncommon in the case of an older man who gradually experiences chronic impotence after many years of successful sexual performance with a life-long partner. In such cases, it is very reasonable to suspect that causes other than psychological are at the root of the problem.

SUMMARY

In summary, many factors can result in impotence. As noted at the beginning of this book, it is now believed that over 80 percent of all cases of persistent erectile failure can be traced to one or more physical causes of the problem. The remaining 20 percent is accounted for by situations where there is a physical cause of undetermined origin or where factors of a purely psychological nature are at work. All factors, even those of a strictly psychological nature, must somehow adversely affect the normal functioning of the blood supply and nervous system serving the penis.

As many cases of impotence go undiagnosed and unreported, there is little hard data on the relative importance in American men of the various physical causes. As a consequence, estimates by authorities differ. Our estimates (shown in the accompanying exhibit) are based upon a consensus of data from published sources. Of course, in many men, multiple causes are at work.

Vascular disease and diabetes appear to be the two most common single causes of erectile dysfunction. Vascular disease, which includes both problems affecting the arterial blood supply to the penis and control of flow in the veins draining blood from the penis, is a consequence of the aging process as programmed into our individual genes and life-style factors such as improper diet, inadequate exercise, and cigarette smoking. This is one area where prevention can play a very important role. Diabetes is a disease that becomes more common with increasing age, but the exact cause is still unknown. We do not as yet know how to prevent diabetes, but effective treatments do exist, including dealing with the resulting erectile dysfunction.[1]

The remaining causes of impotence fall into several diverse categories. Of the group, the possibility of effective prevention is greatest in the case of impotence that is the result of prescription and nonprescription medications and legal and illegal substance abuse.

PHYSICAL IMPOTENCE BY UNDERLYING CAUSE

Cause	Percent
Vascular disease	30
Diabetes Mellitus	30
Drug related[1]	12
Radical prostate and other pelvic surgery	10
Spinal cord and other injuries	10
Endocrine disorders (other than diabetes)	5
Multiple sclerosis	3
Total	100

1 Prescription and over-the-counter drugs as well as substance abuse.

WHEN TO GET HELP—DIAGNOSES THAT YOU CAN DO YOURSELF

Procrastination, unfortunately, is a very common trait in men suffering from any type of sexual dysfunction. In treating erectile dysfunction, in particular, physicians often see individuals who have waited for years before seeking help. And it is a frequent occurrence to hear these patients, overjoyed by their successful treatment, express great regret and even guilt for not having sought help sooner.

Self-recrimination for having procrastinated, however, is not always justified. It is often difficult to know when a problem is serious enough. In individual episodes of impotence, the male partner, of course, is generally quite aware of performance failure. Isolated episodes of impotence, however, are common and do not necessarily show all the signs of being a chronic problem. Just how frequently does failure have to occur before it is reasonable to conclude that help is needed? This is a difficult question to answer. To complicate the situation further, chronic erectile dysfunction often develops gradually, over a period of years, and the ability to perform adequately may ebb and flow while the overall decline is in progress.

Systematic self-evaluation, combined with reliable background information, is critical in making the decision whether or not to seek help. The objective of this chapter is to provide you with sufficient information to conduct this systematic self-evaluation when various types of male sexual dysfunction are suspected. Major emphasis is given to recognizing the problem of impotence, although the self-evaluation of other male sexual dysfunction problems is also included, as well as information on several other male genital problems that are sometimes encountered.

To evaluate your own situation, it is best to keep a simple written record indicating the frequency and extent of performance failure over a period of several months, which you will show to your urologist or other health care professional. The availability of a written record helps overcome embarrassment when discussing problems with a health care professional. It will also prove helpful if you take along a copy of your answers to the questions shown in the accompanying checklist of possible impotence symptoms.

HOW TO RECOGNIZE IMPOTENCE

An episode of impotence may be said to have occurred when the male partner attempts normal vaginal intercourse and is either unable to achieve an erection of sufficient rigidity for penetration or, given penetration, finds that the duration of erection proves inadequate for the mutual satisfaction of both parties. Before concluding that impotence has occurred in a given episode, it is sometimes necessary to consider whether the time was sufficient to permit the achievement of an erection and the orgasmic characteristics of the female partner.

The length of time to achieve an erection can vary considerably for different men. An average man in his midtwenties often experiences an erection in 25 seconds given only visual stimulation, such as the presence of an appealing female partner or the viewing of erotic material. Other men, especially with increasing age, tend to require more time and some degree of physical manipulation. It is reasonable to conclude that failure has occurred when an erection is absent after a period of several minutes, assuming a favorable environment, erotic stimulation, and reasonable manipulation by a cooperative partner.

Your Personal Impotence Checklist

Your Current Sexual Performance

1. Have you been experiencing difficulty recently in achieving erections that you and your partner consider adequate for vaginal intercourse?
2. Does this problem occur three out of every four times or more whenever you attempt intercourse?
3. Do you usually attempt intercourse under favorable conditions, including when well rested, not under the influence of alcohol or other drugs, with suitable privacy, and following adequate erotic stimulation (foreplay)?

Your Recent Sexual Performance Trends

1. For how long have you been experiencing difficulty in achieving adequate erections when attempting intercourse?

2. Are you experiencing erections less frequently than in the past when awaking at night or in the morning or under spontaneous circumstances?

3. How much longer does it take you to achieve erection than in the past?

4. Is the length of time that you can sustain an adequate erection during intercourse noticeably less than in the past?

5. Do you often lose your erection when assuming the position desired by you and your partner for intercourse?

6. Has it become more difficult to have intercourse in certain sexual positions?

7. If you masturbate, do you sometimes ejaculate in the absence of a full erection and has it become more difficult to successfully masturbate in general?

Your Medical Condition

1. Have you ever had a heart attack, stroke, thrombophlebitis (blood clot in the leg or elsewhere), or some other disorder of a cardiovascular nature?

2. Have you ever been told that you have any form of cardiovascular disease, especially heart disease, arteriosclerosis, peripheral vascular disease (PVD), and/or hypertension?

3. Have you ever had an operation for heart disease or some other cardiovascular problem?

4. Have you ever been told that you have an elevated cholesterol level?

5. Do you ever experience serious pain in the legs when walking?

6. Are you taking any form of drug for a cardiovascular problem, especially hypertension?

7. Are you undergoing any form of hormonal therapy, such as that in connection with a benign or malignant prostate tumor?

8. Are you taking drugs on a prescription basis for any other problem?

9. Do you have any known glandular disorder, especially diabetes?

10. Have you experienced a loss of sexual desire (libido) or a general feeling of weakness or malaise?

11. Do you have any known neurological disorder such as multiple sclerosis, Parkinson's disease, or epilepsy?

12. Have you ever had major surgery in the pelvic area, especially surgery involving the prostate gland, bladder, testicles, rectum, anus, and colon?

13. Have you ever had radiation treatment in the pelvic area, especially treatment involving the prostate gland?

14. Have you ever had an injury involving the penis or perineum (hidden portion of the penis), elsewhere in the pelvic area, or in the back, spinal cord, or head?

15. Have you ever had an episode of priapism (persistent longstanding erection)?

16. Does your penis appear to be curved when you have an erection? And does the curvature cause pain to either you or your partner during intercourse?

Your Personal Life-style

1. Do you now smoke or did you once smoke for a long period of time?

2. Are you a heavy drinker or a diagnosed alcoholic?

3. Have you used various illegal drugs, especially cocaine?

4. Are you a frequent user of nonprescription drugs?

5. Are you excessively overweight?

6. Do you exercise regularly?

7. Do you have a close and healthy relationship with your partner (if any)?

It is more difficult to define how long an erection should be maintained after penetration to allow for the mutual satisfaction of both parties. Loss of an erection, accompanied by ejaculation, during penetration or after the first few pelvic thrusts, constitutes premature ejaculation rather than impotence, and is discussed separately. The maintenance of an erection without desired ejaculation for extended periods, perhaps 15 minutes or more, is indicative of ejaculatory failure, or retarded ejaculation, and is also discussed separately. Loss of erection prior to ejaculation, either immediately after penetration or in a relatively short time period, such as 5 minutes or less, is indicative of erectile dysfunction.

The length of time an erection should be maintained in order to provide for the satisfaction of the female partner is also a very complex issue. Women differ widely in their ability to achieve orgasm by simple vaginal intercourse. Some women are able to achieve orgasm rapidly in this manner. Other women find it impossible to achieve an orgasm at all by vaginal intercourse. It is unreasonable to conclude that a man is impotent if he is unable to maintain an erection after penetration for a heroic period of time. An erection is adequate, from a male sexual performance standpoint, if it can be sustained within the vagina for a period of about 10 minutes. The male, of course, has an obligation to assist his partner in achieving orgasm by other means should this period of time prove to be inadequate. In this connection, it is worth remembering that the fingers never get soft.

The decision to seek professional help for suspected impotence should include a variety of factors. To help make this decision, several simple tests are available that can be performed at home. It is possible that a single factor or physical response to any one test may, by itself, be sufficient to provide a definite indication of a condition requiring professional attention. If this should not be the case, the overall pattern should be considered in making a decision.

Review the Pattern of Your Recent Sexual Performance

The systematic evaluation of recent sexual performance is the logical starting point in self-evaluation. Recent performance should be examined, and the number of times that episodes of impotence have taken place should be estimated to the best of your ability. In characterizing any given episode as impotence, the preceding discussion of the nature of erectile dysfunction should be taken into consideration.

Ideally, past performance should be reviewed over a period of several months. Most men, of course, do not normally keep a record of such matters. The analysis, therefore, is inherently subject to a degree of inaccuracy. Involving the female partner may prove useful in improving accuracy. It will also go a long way toward establishing rapport and mutual involvement in finding a solution to your common problem.

You can, of course, keep a log of future sexual activity and then analyze the resulting pattern. The problem with this approach is that for some men, the very procedure of keeping a log introduces an element of performance anxiety that could influence the observed pattern.

In general, when impotence occurs one out of every two times, or 50 percent of the time, given a reasonable number of attempts over a period of about a month, there is strong evidence that chronic impotence exists. Under such circumstances, seeking professional assistance is well justified without any further analysis. At the level of one out of every four encounters, or 25 percent of the time, there is a strong possibility of a chronic condition. However, you should consider other factors before seeking assistance. A one-out-of-ten failure level is little reason for immediate concern.

Before concluding that you have experienced an impotence episode, it is important to take into consideration the concept of the "refractory period," the period of time it takes a man following ejaculation to again obtain an erection. In teenagers and young men, the refractory period can often be only a matter of a few minutes. As you grow older, it is quite natural for this to be no longer the case. In general, it would be a mistake for an older man to record as an episode of impotence the failure to achieve an erection during a 24-hour period following ejaculation.

Trends in Sexual Performance

The tendency for impotence to develop gradually over a period of time, especially in the case of older men, makes it highly advisable to evaluate, as objectively as possible, how your recent sexual behavior compares with that of past years. The onset of impotence very frequently takes place over a two- to five-year period. During this time, an awareness of the condition gradually emerges. For this reason, going back for a period of about five years is particularly relevant for older men who first become suspicious of a possible impotence condition.

Recalling accurately the frequency of sexual intercourse and the extent of performance failure over a long period of time is very difficult. Fortunately, you can get a good idea of what has been happening by evaluating these four conditions:

◆ Frequency of erections when awakening in the morning or at night or spontaneously at other times

◆ Length of time required to initiate and obtain a full erection

◆ Your ability to assume varied sexual positions

◆ The length of time an erection is typically sustained

Virtually every healthy young man experiences the presence of a full erection immediately upon awakening from sleep in the morning and often when awakening during the night. The presence of such an erection is normal and is related to the frequent erections that occur unconsciously during sleep. As a condition of chronic impotence becomes established, the frequency of firmness of morning erections diminishes. The total absence of such erections is a strong indication of chronic impotence, usually of a physical origin.

Men who are recovering from various types of major surgery sometimes report the absence of erections upon awakening and often express concern. In cases where such men do not have a chronic impotence condition, normal erectile performance usually returns in time, and the return of function suggests a proper progression of the recovery process.

Spontaneous erections occur during waking hours and in the absence of physical stimulation. Such erections are often noticed by younger men when viewing erotic material, or even in casual conversation with attractive women. When spontaneous erections no longer occur in men for whom such erections were previously common, there is a reasonable suggestion of some loss of sexual vigor.

As previously mentioned, with increasing age men usually require more stimulation to achieve erections. Such change can be gradual. A significant change in a relatively short period of time, however, suggests the development of chronic impotence.

A very revealing symptom at the onset of chronic impotence is the increasing inability to assume varied positions during sexual intercourse. Certain men, because of social conditioning or religious beliefs, rarely attempt intercourse in any manner other than the familiar "missionary" position. In the case of a man who has regularly employed different positions, and now finds that intercourse in only one position is possible, there is good indication of an evolving impotence problem, most likely related to changes that have been taking place in the vascular system.

The term "steal syndrome" is used for a particular frustrating problem in which erections occur in the resting state but are rapidly lost after assuming the desired position for intercourse, either immediately following vaginal penetration or following the first few pelvic thrusts. The term refers to the fact that as the level of sexual activity increases, blood is "stolen" from the penis and pelvic area, resulting in the loss of erection. The problem is believed to be largely due to a narrowing of both of the internal iliac arteries serving the pelvic area. As a result, blood is diverted away from the corpora cavernosa to the vascular system serving the gluteal area (buttocks). It may be in some men that the steal syndrome takes place only when certain positions are attempted. Often a change of position, such as the woman on top, may result in improved performance.

Another revealing trend in sexual performance is the inability to maintain a firm erection for an extended period of time. In some instances, this may indicate that the steal syndrome is at work. It may also be indicative of a leakage problem in which the smooth muscles within the penis are incapable of retaining sufficient blood within the corpora cavernosa.

Self-evaluation Tests You Can Do at Home

Masturbation Performance

The ability to masturbate successfully, with a full erection, constitutes a test for chronic impotence that can be easily performed at home. When attempted, there are several possible outcomes:

- There is an absence of both erection and ejaculation.
- Ejaculation takes place in the absence of an erection.
- Both full erection and ejaculation take place.
- Full erection is achieved, but ejaculation does not take place.

When masturbation, performed under suitable conditions, consistently results in neither erection nor ejaculation, chronic impotence of a physical nature is strongly indicated. In Western culture, however, a strong religious and social taboo has historically existed against masturbation. As a consequence, it is possible that some individuals find it virtually impossible to achieve an erection from self-stimulation. In either case, any individual who cannot obtain an erection from self-stimulation, or has no recollection of ever having an erection, is well-advised to seek professional help.

It is quite possible for a man to masturbate to ejaculation despite the absence of an erection, or to ejaculate with an erection of insufficient firmness for vaginal penetration. Chronic impotence is most likely present in such individuals, and professional help should be sought. Because the ability to ejaculate successfully suggests the absence of a psychological barrier against masturbation, it's quite likely that the impotence has physical causes.

When a man who has been experiencing impotence symptoms during sexual intercourse is able to masturbate successfully to ejaculation with a full erection, psychological impotence is a definite possibility. It is possible, however, that the condition has a physical origin. For example, the problem may again be the steal syndrome: the limited physical activities associated with masturbation are not sufficient to result in loss of erection, in contrast with the increased sexual activity that occurs during regular intercourse and that results in loss of erection. Regardless of the origin of the problem, professional attention is definitely indicated for men who can successfully masturbate and ejaculate with full erection, but consistently prove impotent during sexual relations with a partner.

The final masturbation possibility, erection without ejaculation, indicates the dysfunction known as ejaculatory failure. An individual who can achieve erection through masturbation, but cannot ejaculate, is usually capable of vaginal penetration.

Postage Stamp Test

Nocturnal erections occur in periods known as rapid eye movement (REM) sleep, in intervals typically 5 to 30 minutes long, during which dreams usually occur. While in the REM state, it is highly unlikely that psychological factors can prevent erections in a man physically capable of having an erection.

In the professional investigation of impotence, an electronic monitoring instrument is sometimes used to determine the incidence of nocturnal erections. During the test, a sensor is attached to the penis to monitor and record changes in penis size.

It is possible to obtain a reasonable approximation of the test with only a coil of perforated U.S. postage stamps.

For economy, use of one-cent stamps is suggested. Prior to retiring for the evening, simply encircle the soft penis with a sufficient number of stamps to form a ring. Moisten the back of one of the end stamps. Overlap the face of the stamp at the other end of the ring and hold the ring in place long enough to stick.

Immediately after awakening the next morning, examine the stamps. If the ring is broken at any one of the perforations, it means that at least one erection did occur during the night. (The postage stamp test, of course, will not reveal whether there has been more than one erection, as can be done with the more complicated medical device. It also will not reveal whether or not the erect penis would have had sufficient rigidity to permit vaginal penetration or whether the erection would have been of sufficient duration for successful intercourse.)

If the postage stamp test, however, reveals the absence of a nocturnal erection, there is very good indication of chronic impotence of a physical origin. If an erection did take place, impotence of a psychological or physical nature is still a possibility.

Simple Neurological Tests

Three simple tests can be performed at home, by yourself or with a partner, which provide clues to the functioning of the neurological system of the penis and pelvic area. The first, known as the cremasteric reflex test, measures the adequacy of the neural connections to the pelvic area. To perform this test, lie on your back, then either you or your partner should make a light quick stroke with a blunt pointed object across several inches of the inner side of your upper thigh. The normal response is a quick upward movement of the testicle on the same side of the body where the stroke was made. The lack of such movement on either side of the body indicates the possibility of a neurological problem in the spinal column or brain. Professional investigation is recommended both for the treatment of impotence as well as for general health.

As all healthy men living outside the tropics know, the scrotum will tighten up and draw upward into the body when exposed to low temperature conditions. This response is part of the normal mechanism used to maintain seminal fluid at the proper temperature for reproductive purposes. In the ice-cube test, an ice cube or some other very cold object is placed momentarily on the scrotum. The normal response should be a rapid, easily observed contraction. Lack of this response indicates a neurological problem warranting professional investigation.

The final test is for the more adventurous, but actually it can be performed easily. The bulbocavernosus (BC) reflex test involves the insertion of a finger in the anus and the simultaneous quick squeezing of the tip of the penis. If the neurological system is functioning properly, a quick contraction in the rectal area should be felt.

Simple Vascular Tests

Several simple home tests or observations can be made that provide clues to the possible existence of vascular or blood flow problems possibly related to impotence. The results of these tests or observations are by themselves not conclusive, but they may indicate an overall pattern.

The first is a simple walking test. To perform this test, merely walk a distance of at least one mile at a fairly fast pace. While overexertion should be avoided, the pace and distance should be both faster and somewhat longer than usual. Of course, caution is advised for individuals with known cardiovascular problems. If a fairly piercing pain is noted in either or both calves, evidence exists of an oxygen insufficiency and impaired blood flow to the lower portion of the body. While the walking test does not directly indicate impaired blood flow to the penis, it is a good indication of the possibility. Should you experience significant pain when performing the walking test, it would be a good idea to bring this to the attention of your physician, in view of its general implications as to your cardiovascular health.

Examination of the genital area may also yield significant evidence of possible vascular problems. When the penis is found to be consistently cold, even when exposed to warm temperatures, there is a possibility of vascular insufficiency. Abnormalities in the color of the penis are also an important indication of vascular insufficiency. In men with light-colored skin, the penis may take on a distinct blue color when blood flow is impaired. The effect is not as easy to detect with dark-skinned men, but a definite difference in appearance may be noted.

A final observation concerns the presence of firm, hard areas in the penis. Such areas are typically found along both sides of the penis, in the general area where the penis is attached to the body. It is not uncommon to encounter patients at the urologist's office who have noticed hard areas of the penis and are fearful of cancer. Such hard areas, however, usually result from the calcification of the corporal bodies (blood-carrying bodies) in the penis due to the gradual accumulation of plaque. The resulting restriction in blood flow can cause erection difficulties.

While examining your genital area for indications of vascular problems, it would be a good idea to take a moment and feel through your scrotum for any possible abnormality such as a lump or a testicle that seems larger than usual. Doing so might just provide early warning of testicular cancer.

Review Your Medical History

A thorough self-evaluation should include the careful analysis of your personal medical history, particularly with respect to specific health problems known to be linked with impotence. It is especially important to try to relate the onset of any known impotence-linked problem with the first appearance of significant impotence symptoms.

In reviewing your medical history, the preliminary medical history questionnaire shown in Appendix B to this book should prove useful. This questionnaire is completed by all new patients at the Morganstern Urology Clinic, Atlanta, Georgia. Take a copy of the filled-out questionnaire with you, should you consult a urologist for a male sexual dysfunction problem or, for that matter, any other health care provider regarding any type of medical problem.

The following list summarizes the important factors of your medical history that you should consider when performing a self-evaluation in connection with possible erectile dysfunction:

◆ Cardiovascular diseases

◆ Diabetes mellitus

◆ Endocrine (glandular) problems, other than diabetes

◆ Neurological disorders

◆ Pelvic surgery and radiation therapy

◆ Accidents to the head, spinal cord, and pelvic area

◆ Exposure to known environmental hazards

Men with a history that includes some type of cardiovascular disease should definitely be aware of a possible link with impotence. This is especially true for individuals with heart disease, blood vessel disease, or hypertension or those who have experienced coronary artery bypass surgery. A history of any of these problems, combined with frequent impotence episodes and any possible symptoms observed in the simple vascular tests, strongly indicates the need to seek professional assistance.

Given the strong link between impotence and diabetes, any man with a known case of diabetes should be on the lookout for impotence symptoms, and should be prepared to seek assistance, even if such symptoms have not yet appeared. It is a primary responsibility of any physician treating a diabetes patient to explain the possible sexual ramifications of the disease and to encourage consultation with specialists on sexual dysfunction when indicated. All older men should be on the lookout for possible diabetes symptoms, as the disease often occurs later in life in marginal form and may take a while to be detected. A real warning sign would be a combination of impotence, renal (kidney), and retinal (eye) problems.

Individuals with known glandular disorders, other than diabetes, should consider the possibility of a connection with any impotence symptoms that are being experienced. This is particularly true should you have a history of pituitary and adrenal gland disorders. Men with known problems of the testicles, particularly those associated with inadequate testosterone production, should also be prepared to seek professional attention when impotence symptoms are noted. The same advice applies to men with known problems of the thyroid. When there are no known glandular problems, the presence of extreme obesity, chronic fatigue, breast enlargement and other feminine characteristics, and erectile dysfunction can be an indication that such problems may very well exist.

Neurological disorders are generally believed to be of lesser importance as underlying causes of impotence than cardiovascular disease or diabetes. Men with known nervous system disorders, including epilepsy, Parkinson's disease, and multiple sclerosis, however, should be aware of the possible connection, and are advised to seek professional help when experiencing impotence symptoms. Impotence is also linked to various types of brain tumors, which is another good reason not to neglect the presence of persistent impotence symptoms.

Any man who has experienced major surgery or radiation therapy in the pelvic region, especially procedures involving the prostate gland, anus, rectum, bladder, and colon, should seek professional help if impotence symptoms are experienced. Usually, impotence shows up fairly soon after such procedures, although the onset of the problem can be delayed. Men scheduled for such surgery should always discuss the possibility of impotence in advance with their physician, in the hope that a problem can be avoided or at least minimized.

Individuals who have experienced accidental injuries to the head, spinal cord, and pelvic area are also advised to obtain professional help whenever frequent impotence episodes are noted. It would be helpful to ask the parents or other relatives of a patient about his past injuries or accidents because major childhood injuries, which the patient may have completely forgotten, can be a cause of adult impotence. This can be the case especially with injuries that took place to young boys while they were in a straddle position, such as when riding a bicycle. Straddle injuries can be particularly serious as sharp blows to the perineum (crotch) and the pelvic bone may result in damage to the arteries supplying blood to the penis or scar erectile tissues in that portion of the penis inside the body.

Environmental health is an increasingly important medical specialty. If you were exposed to any known environmental hazard as a child or have worked in occupations where there has been a chance of exposure to toxic chemicals or radiation, you should note this in your self-evaluation. A partial list of hazardous materials that may be encountered on the job include lead, mercury, cadmium, beryllium, pesticides, and industrial solvents. Exposure to hazardous materials and radiation can result in impotence due to nerve damage, although the possibility does exist of damage to internal organs, which, in turn, may contribute to erectile dysfunction. Lead poisoning can be particularly damaging to the peripheral nervous system. Lead-based paints are no longer permitted for inside use, but the possibility exists for exposure, especially to children raised in older homes.

Review Your Use of Prescription and Nonprescription Drugs

The link between impotence and many frequently used medications is discussed in Chapter 4, along with a listing of many of the problem drugs currently in use today. It is important to recognize that because new drugs are constantly being introduced in the pharmaceutical field, no listing of problem drugs will ever be complete. Therefore, if a drug you are taking or plan to take is not included in the list in Chapter 4, that is no guarantee that the drug is free of problems. Fortunately, many newer drugs are much improved with respect to impotence and other side effects, but that is not always the case. If information on any drug that you are taking or will be taking has not been provided by your regular physician, you would be well advised to consult the latest edition of the *Physicians' Desk Reference* published annually by Medical Economics Company, Oradell, New Jersey. This book, commonly known as the *"PDR,"* is usually found at better public libraries. The contents of the PDR are now also on computer and your physician may have access through a data network. *The Physicians' Desk Reference for Nonprescription Drugs,* by the same publisher, provides information on the side effects of over-the-counter products.

The American Urological Association (AUA) has in the past published a listing of drugs linked to sexual dysfunction. The most recent listing, unfortunately, is now about ten years old. You could check the AUA to see if anything is known regarding any newer drug that you may be taking. The address of this organization, and of several other organizations that provide information on problem drugs, is given in Appendix C.

Any man who has been using a prescription drug linked to impotence should not immediately discontinue its use upon becoming aware of that fact. This sometimes happens, particularly in the case of men using medications for high blood pressure. Such men, of course, subject themselves to the long-term danger of strokes, heart attacks, and other problems. With some drugs, precipitous withdrawal can present a very real and immediate danger. The best course of action is to first talk with the physician who has prescribed the suspected drug. Sometimes an alternative medication is available, with lesser side effects. Should your physician be unresponsive, get a second opinion before discontinuing the drug.

Inventory Your Alcohol, Tobacco, and Illegal Drug Use

Any man who is a heavy drinker or is a diagnosed alcoholic should be aware of the strong possibility of impotence and should not hesitate to seek help, even when relatively infrequent episodes of impotence are first experienced. Moderate social drinking, however, is not grounds for seeking immediate help, unless an impotence problem is becoming chronic and other contributory problems are observed in self-evaluation.

Infrequent use of illegal substances, including marijuana and cocaine, in itself is not sufficient reason to conclude that immediate professional attention is required after a few impotence episodes. Heavy users of such substances, however, are advised to seek professional treatment for both impotence and drug dependency, even after a relatively small number of impotence episodes.

As discussed, smoking tobacco tends to decrease the flow of blood throughout the vascular system, and specifically in the penile artery. Cigarette smokers experiencing symptoms should consider trying the simple vascular tests described previously. If these tests reveal the possible presence of a vascular problem, it would be a good idea to obtain help even after a relatively small number of impotence episodes.

There is increasing evidence of the dangers of secondary tobacco smoke. The area is controversial, with cigarette manufacturers currently denying that secondary smoke constitutes a hazard to nonsmokers. Should you live with a smoker or your occupation necessitates exposure to secondary smoke, especially in situations where air is continuously recycled, you would be well advised to try the indicated simple vascular tests.

HOW TO RECOGNIZE SEXUAL DYSFUNCTION PROBLEMS OTHER THAN IMPOTENCE

The accompanying table provides a summary of male dysfunction problems. The common definitions shown in the table should prove useful in clearly stating the nature of your problem, should the need for help be indicated. Of course, it is possible to experience a combination of dysfunction problems.

SUMMARY OF MALE SEXUAL DYSFUNCTION PROBLEMS

Problem	Common Definition
Impotence	The inability to achieve an erection of sufficient rigidity for vaginal penetration or of sufficient duration for the mutual satisfaction of both partners.
Premature Ejaculation	A condition in which a man lacks adequate voluntary control over the length of time to reach ejaculation as reasonably desired by both sexual partners.
Retrograde Ejaculation	Ejaculation usually taking place with adequate physical sensation, but without the normal flow of ejaculatory fluid from the tip of the penis. The fluid backs up into the bladder and subsequently passes harmlessly out of the body during normal urination.
Ejaculatory Failure	The inability to ejaculate within a reasonable period of time or not at all, despite the ability to achieve and maintain an adequate erection.
Priapism	Painful and unwanted erections that continue for extended periods of time.
Peyronie's Disease	A condition characterized by a penis that, when erect, is bent out of shape, with the curvature often causing pain and discomfort to one or both sexual partners during intercourse.
Painful Ejaculation	Pain or abnormal discomfort experienced during ejaculation.
Lack of Desire	The complete, or nearly complete, abnormal absence of sexual interest (libido).
Performance Anxiety	The abnormal fear of engaging in sexual activities.
Prostate Irritation	Pain and discomfort experienced in the vicinity of the prostate, resulting from a man's pattern of sexual behavior.
Unretractable Foreskin	A condition in which a man is unable to pull the foreskin back over the head of the penis.

Premature Ejaculation

Ejaculation that frequently takes place well before it is desired by either sexual partner is considered premature. Some men with the problem will ejaculate spontaneously during foreplay, or very shortly after first being touched in the genital area. Most men with the problem, however, ejaculate during vaginal penetration, but after only the first few pelvic thrusts. Premature ejaculation should not be confused with the inability of a man to voluntarily avoid ejaculation for an unreasonably extended period, especially with a woman who requires an extended period to achieve an orgasm or supplemental stimulation.

It is a popular belief that premature ejaculation is almost always a problem experienced by sexually naive younger men in early sexual encounters. The extraordinary level of arousal that is supposed to occur under such circumstances presumably causes almost instantaneous erection and ejaculation. Mild versions of the supposedly comical and usually humiliating event have on occasion been portrayed on the stage and screen.

Jeff, a 38-year-old financial executive, began to experience premature ejaculation with his wife after 15 years of marriage. His problem was complicated by guilt over a recent extramarital affair. He reasoned that his problem was somehow due to an excess of ardor brought on by the need to compensate for his feelings of guilt.

While premature ejaculation may have a psychological cause, it can also have a physical origin. The problem may frequently occur in men with infections of the prostate. In such cases, the problem usually makes its appearance shortly after the onset of the infection. Examination revealed that Jeff had an inflamed prostate. The premature ejaculation condition disappeared after treatment. The link between premature ejaculation and prostate infections makes it logical to regard premature ejaculation as a possible symptom of a prostate infection.

To determine if a premature ejaculation problem exists, you should first record how often you have experienced the symptom. As with impotence, a period of at least one month should be examined. It is reasonable to seek professional help when the problem occurs during approximately one out of every four sexual encounters, or about 25 percent of the time.

Before seeking help, it would be a good idea to examine yourself for indications of an inflamed prostate. These include

◆ A penile discharge of a generally white appearance

◆ Ejaculate which appears bloody

◆ Burning sensation when urinating

◆ Unusually frequent urination at night

◆ Restricted flow during urination and frequent stopping and starting of the urinary stream during urination

The simple examination of the prostate that is typically performed in a routine physical examination is generally not enough to diagnose a prostatic infection capable of causing premature ejaculation. A vigorous massage of the prostate by a urological specialist and the laboratory examination of expelled prostatic fluid are required.

Retrograde Ejaculation

In retrograde ejaculation, there is impaired flow of ejaculatory fluid from the tip of the penis. Although retrograde ejaculation does not normally reduce the sexual pleasure to either partner, it is an obvious problem when children are desired. The condition occurs when the sphincter muscle that usually shuts off the passageway through which urine travels from the bladder to the penis during periods of sexual activity fails to function properly. When this happens, ejaculatory fluid backs up into the bladder. Subsequently, the fluid passes harmlessly out of the body during normal urination. Retrograde ejaculation, however, should not be counted on for birth control purposes as there sometimes can be movement of semen through the penis sufficient to result in pregnancy.

Damage to the sphincter can be caused by routine prostate surgery, damage to the nerves at the base of the bladder, and spinal cord injury. Another cause is diabetes and for this reason, especially, the condition should not be neglected. Retrograde ejaculation has also been linked to Mellaril (thioridazine), a drug used in the treatment of emotional problems.

It may be some time before the existence of a retrograde ejaculation problem is observed, as the feeling of ejaculation continues even in the absence of ejaculate. A slight cloudy condition seen in the first urination following intercourse may be the first symptom. Should this be seen, it is, of course, possible to check for the presence of ejaculate in the vagina of the partner. The absence of ejaculate in the vagina, however, is not always obvious. Masturbation represents the conclusive test for the condition.

Ejaculatory Failure

Ejaculatory failure, or the failure to ejaculate, is fortunately a relatively rare condition, as it is difficult to treat. The definitive cause of the problem has yet to be satisfactorily determined, but there is evidence that both psychological and physical factors may play a role.

Masters and Johnson studies have suggested that the problem is largely psychological, and occurs most often in men with very sexually inhibiting religious and moral backgrounds. Theresa Larsen Crenshaw, M.D., a sex therapist based in southern California, has observed that the overwhelming number of men who report the problem are from Jewish backgrounds. This has not always been found to be the case, however. In Atlanta, a metropolitan area with a relatively low Jewish population, ejaculatory failure shows up as frequently in patients as elsewhere.

If ejaculatory failure were to be demonstrated to be a problem highly characteristic of Jewish men, one possible explanation might be cultural attitudes that result in psychological barriers to sexual performance. Inhibiting attitudes toward sexual matters exist among traditional Jews, as in most traditional cultures. This does not seem to have prevented the existence of the very large families characteristic of the fundamentalist sect known as the Hasidim.

Another explanation might be the religious practice of circumcision common to both the Jewish and Islamic traditions. Circumcision does somewhat decrease the sensitivity of the tip of the penis, with conceivable psychological or physical consequences. The problem with this explanation is that most American men have been routinely circumcised since the 1940s. At present about 80 percent of all American males are circumcised, although the operation is rarely a medical necessity. If circumcision was the root cause of ejaculatory failure, the problem would obviously be far more common.

The consistent inability to ejaculate within a period of 15 minutes or even more, despite the presence of a firm erection and suitable surroundings, is indicative of ejaculatory failure. When failure occurs 25 percent of the time or more, professional help is indicated.

Ejaculatory failure has been linked to a number of drugs used for the control of emotional problems, cardiovascular disorders, and prostate tumors. These drugs are listed in Appendix A. As discussed in Chapter 3, there is also some evidence that a class of naturally occurring chemical substances known as prostaglandins may play a role in ejaculation. This might suggest that the absence of prostaglandins or the presence of other substances that may interfere with prostaglandins could be a factor in ejaculatory failure.

When the problem is experienced with one partner, but not another, or when the man subject to the problem is able to successfully masturbate, it is reasonable to assume that psychological factors are at work. The presence of the problem, combined with the inability to masturbate successfully, tends to indicate an increased likelihood of a physical problem, although this is not always the case.

Priapism

Priapism derives its name from the minor Greek god Priapus. The deity was portrayed in antiquity by a figure with an enormous, constantly erect phallus (penis). Despite the many tall tales told by "studs," supererections that last for hours are not an everyday occurrence, or anything to be admired.

Priapism is a serious condition that should receive immediate medical attention, regardless of any embarrassment. The danger is that the extended interruption of the supply of oxygen and other constituents of the blood to the penis that occurs in priapism can result in extensive internal damage to the penis, rendering the normal erection mechanism inoperative.

During an incident of priapism, the blood becomes sludgelike, a condition that can directly cause impotence due to the blockage of blood flow. The condition can occur in cancer. Also, an erection suggestive of priapism may occur during penile injection therapy, when papaverine or other drugs are being used to promote erection. Several drugs have been linked to priapism (see Appendix A).

Distinguishing an erection due to priapism from a normal erection is usually not too difficult. Any erection that persists without continuing physical stimulation for more than one-half hour, and is not relieved through ejaculation or negative thought processes, is suspect, unless erections of this duration have been common in the past. In priapism, erections can actually last for several days, but help should be obtained after an unwanted erection continues for more than several hours. Erections obtained during penile injection therapy in an impotence treatment program under a urologist's direction normally last one to two hours. Chapter 7 discusses what to expect and what you should do in this type of treatment.

Peyronie's Disease

Peyronie's disease, or the bent penis syndrome, is caused by the formation of scar tissue along the walls of the erectile chambers of the penis. The condition was first described by François de la Peyronie, a physician in the court of Louis XIV of France. This scarring results from plaque deposits and, in time, results in bending the penis in the direction of the side of the penis where the scarring is most severe.

Peyronie's disease most often occurs, without any obvious reason, in men age 40 and older, although cases have been reported in teenagers. About 1 percent of all men in the most vulnerable age group are reported to experience the disorder. The disease sometimes occurs in men who are heavy users of alcohol. At times, the symptoms of the disease disappear on their own. In almost one-third of the cases, the disease results in significant penile deformity and painful erection. In some cases, an erection may occur at the rear of the penis, beyond the point of maximum plaque buildup, but not at the front or downstream end. Often, the deformity and pain it causes during erection may be sufficient to make vaginal penetration difficult, if not impossible.

Peyronie's disease should be suspected and help obtained whenever there has been a noticeable change in the shape of the erect penis. The condition usually develops over a period of time, and is often overlooked until painful erection makes vaginal penetration difficult.

Just as women are advised to perform periodic breast self-examination, it is a good idea for all men to regularly check the general condition of their penis. A sign of possible Peyronie's disease is a buildup of scar tissue that can be felt beneath the skin of a nonerect penis as a hard nodule. Pain experienced by either partner during intercourse is another possible sign of the disease.

Painful Ejaculation

The sensations of pleasure and pain are, to a degree, interconnected in the brain and nervous system. As a consequence, it may be difficult to distinguish low levels of pain from pleasure during ejaculation. The difficulty is compounded by the obvious preoccupation of the man during sexual intercourse. At more intense levels of discomfort, however, a painful condition should become quite obvious. Painful ejaculation can actually extend to a point where sexual activities are precluded.

There are various causes of painful ejaculation. The most common problem is an infection of the prostate and/or one or both of the seminal vesicles. If there is any doubt that pain is being felt, masturbation represents a good way to check. Persistent pain should be investigated professionally, especially if other symptoms are apparent, such as unusual penile discharges.

Lack of Desire

Sexual interest, or libido, is a very normal characteristic of all healthy males beyond the age of puberty. Sexual interest, of course, is held in check by social convention, moral convictions, and the legal system. The lack of sexual desire, even in an individual who, for religious purposes, has taken a vow of chastity, is abnormal, and may be symptomatic of an underlying physical problem. In the marital situation, lack of desire can often weaken or damage the marital relationship.

Possible physical causes of lack of desire include hyperthyroidism and kidney problems. Anything, such as alcoholism, that depresses testosterone or increases estrogen production can result in lack of desire. A fairly lengthy list of drugs used for the treatment of emotional problems, prostate tumors, alcoholism, and cardiovascular and gastrointestinal disorders have been linked to loss of desire (see Appendix A).

Men with a lack of sexual desire are not always aware of the condition. Often, the matter is first mentioned by the partner. If lack of desire becomes apparent in a stable relationship between two partners, it is helpful to observe whether certain physical conditions often associated with lack of desire are apparent, such as chronic fatigue, general malaise, and depression. Such symptoms may indicate hyperthyroidism. It is also advisable to investigate any change that may be noticed in the size and shape of the testicles, allowing for the possibility of some impairment in testosterone production. Professional help should be obtained whenever lack of desire persists for several months or is combined with the other symptoms noted previously.

Performance Anxiety

Performance anxiety is characterized by the abnormal fear of sexual activities in a man whose libido remains at normal levels. A man experiencing this condition may consciously or unconsciously avoid contact with potential sexual partners or avoid sexual relations with an existing partner.

In the past, performance anxiety has generally been considered essentially a psychological problem caused by such factors as guilt, fear of punishment, and fear of possible ridicule by a sexual partner. As noted in Chapter 1, the popular belief that the feminist movement, characterized by more sexually aware and demanding women, has resulted in the increased incidence of performance anxiety problems in men is not supported by scientific evidence.

Psychological explanations of performance anxiety do not adequately account for problems of this nature that may arise in older men, who have successfully engaged in sexual activities for many years, typically with a long-time partner. In such cases, the underlying cause of performance anxiety may be the onset of impotence brought on by one or more very real physical problems. Performance anxiety problems may be triggered in some men by premature ejaculation resulting from a physical cause.

Performance anxiety is easily detected when obvious symptoms such as panic, fear, increased pulse rate, and hyperventilation take place before and during a sexual situation. The problem is more difficult to detect in a man who unconsciously avoids sexual contacts. The persistence of obvious symptoms indicates a need for professional help. Adult males who are aware of a strong desire for sex, but deliberately avoid the sexual act, should also seek help. This, of course, does not apply to men who are obligated or required to be celibate.

Prostate Irritation

Prostate irritation is a condition characterized by pain and tenderness in the vicinity of the prostate and genital organs.

Although the pain is typically mild and usually disappears in a few hours, in some men it can cause considerable discomfort and become chronic in nature. A man's pattern of sexual activity can be the cause of the problem.

Irritation can be experienced when there is an excessive build up of fluid (congestion) inside the prostate gland. This can be the result of lengthy periods of sexual abstinence, extended sexual stimulus not relieved by ejaculation, repeated ejaculatory failure, avoiding ejaculation for lengthy periods to prolong intercourse, and use of coitus interruptus (pulling out) as a form of birth control. Irritation can also be caused when very frequent ejaculations result in strain and fatigue to the semen-producing mechanism of the prostate. This can especially be the case when a sudden increase in sexual activity follows an extended period of sexual abstinence.

Unretractable Penile Foreskin

In infants, the fold of skin at the head of the penis known as the foreskin is normally connected to the tissues of the penis. Usually, starting at about 6 months, the tissues quite naturally start to separate. When a young boy is about 5 years old, the separation is complete, allowing for full retraction of the foreskin, thus facilitating proper hygiene.

In a small number of cases, proper separation fails to occur. The result can be a foreskin that is so tight that it prevents erection. This was the unfortunate dysfunction experienced by Louis VI of France as noted in Chapter 1. An unretractable foreskin, of course, is only a problem experienced by an uncircumcised man.

HOW TO RECOGNIZE OTHER MALE URINARY-GENITAL SYSTEM PROBLEMS

There are a number of other problems that can affect the male urinary-genital system. While these do not always have immediate implications with respect to successful sexual performance, they should not be ignored due to their general health consequences and possible contribution to a dysfunction problem in the long term. In some cases, these problems may also compromise the health of the partner.

Blood in the Urine

Blood in the urine is a serious symptom that deserves prompt professional attention. This advice applies equally to men and women. Possible underlying problems of a serious nature include kidney and bladder tumors. Less serious problems may include various bacterial or viral infections of the bladder, kidney and urethra.

Detecting blood in the urine is usually not difficult. At times, urine can take on an unusual color that may be mistaken for blood, due to the presence of dyes originating in the diet or in medications. For example, urine may take on an orange-red color after taking Azo-Gantrisin and Pyridium. If there is any doubt in such a situation, it is best to promptly seek professional attention. Small quantities of blood in the urine are difficult to detect visually but do show up in standard urinalysis procedures.

Penile Discharges

An unusual penile discharge should be investigated. A whitish discharge, not ejaculate, generally indicates urethritis or a prostate infection. In the former category, chlamydia infections are the most common today. Bloody ejaculate usually results from a prostate infection. Hematospermia is a condition in which large quantities of blood appear to be present in the seminal fluid following ejaculation. The condition can be very alarming to patients, but it is usually not as serious as it looks.

A yellowish discharge, usually accompanied by a burning sensation and frequent urination, can indicate gonorrhea, although other causes are possible. Men noticing this symptom have an obvious responsibility to discontinue sexual activity and to advise sexual partners of the possibility of a problem.

Penile Skin Disorders

Any unusual condition on the skin of the penis that persists for more than a few days deserves professional attention. This includes sores, lumps, and encrusted deposits. In all cases, it is advisable to discontinue sexual activity until the problem is resolved.

Sores and lumps on the penis can indicate various sexually transmitted diseases, such as syphilis and genital herpes. Encrusted deposits may be linked to sexual activities with a partner subject to certain types of vaginitis. When genital herpes proves to be the problem, future sexual activity is possible, but should take place only under suitable circumstances. Intercourse is generally safe during periods when sores are not active in either partner. When a vaginal infection is discovered in the female partner, intercourse should be discontinued until the problem is treated in both partners. Unless this is done, the possibility exists of passing the infection back and forth indefinitely.

Warts on the penis are caused by a virus. The condition does not usually cause a problem to the man. Penile warts, however, should also be promptly treated as there is evidence that they are a factor in triggering cervical cancer in women who engage in intercourse with men with the condition.

Painful and Frequent Urination

Painful urination, similar to painful ejaculation, may indicate a prostate infection. Painful urination may also indicate kidney stones or tumors in the urinary system. All persistent pain should be investigated. Excessive or frequent urination, often accompanied by excessive thirst, can be a symptom of diabetes. This symptom can also indicate possible benign or malignant prostate tumors and certain types of bladder infections. In the case of men with prostate tumors, the urge to urinate frequently may also be accompanied by a period of hesitation before voiding begins, a weak urinary stream, and a feeling of incompleteness following voiding. These symptoms are all the result of the prostate tumor exerting pressure on the urethra.

SUMMARY

Knowing when to get help for a suspected male sexual dysfunction problem requires systematic self-evaluation. It also requires a feeling of commitment on your part, a healthy curiosity as to how your body works, and, ideally, the support of your partner.

After conscientiously applying the information provided in this chapter, you should be able to discern whether or not you have an impotence problem or some other dysfunctional condition of sufficient seriousness to require professional attention. If you determine that you do not need professional help, your effort will still have been worthwhile, in view of what you have learned about the functioning of your body. You will also be prepared for what may develop in the future.

Should you need professional help, the next chapter on sources of help will be of immediate assistance. The information you accumulated in your self-evaluation, especially if recorded on paper, is the type of information you will need to discuss your condition intelligently with a physician.

CHAPTER 6

WHERE TO GET HELP—AND WHAT TO EXPECT

You have carefully followed the suggestions of the previous chapter and have reason to believe that some physical problems exist. You are now faced with a major problem: finding effective help. If you live in a typical large urban center, you must make an essentially uninformed choice between a large number of individual health care providers. Unfortunately, few communities enjoy an efficient referral system for finding a suitable physician. You should be concerned about the degree of understanding and professional capability of any practitioner selected at random from the telephone book. Normally, in seeking a physician, you would ask the advice of friends and acquaintances. But understandably, many people are reluctant to do this when the problem is a sexual dysfunction.

113

This chapter is intended to provide you with a systematic approach to obtaining help. It will also tell you what you should expect and where things can go wrong.

The logical place to start, even if your self-evaluation suggests your problem is psychological in nature, is with a physician familiar with the physical causes of impotence and other male sexual problems. Given the current state of the art, there is virtually no objective way to make a direct diagnosis of psychological impotence. Basically, it is not possible to conclude that psychological impotence exists until all symptoms and known medical problems associated with physical impotence are shown conclusively, by physical examination, not to be present. Failure to eliminate physical impotence as a possibility could result in costly and fruitless psychological treatment or sex therapy. The danger also exists that a potentially dangerous physical problem could go undetected for an extended period.

HOW YOUR REGULAR PHYSICIAN CAN HELP YOU

If a truly efficient system for the delivery of medical services existed, all of us would have convenient and continuing access to a personal physician. Such a physician would be a highly experienced generalist, with a working knowledge of all aspects of medicine and an ongoing familiarity with the medical background of all regular patients. The physician would not be expected to be an expert in every area of medical specialization, but rather an expert on screening medical problems and on preliminary diagnosis. The physician would also be in a position to access rapidly computerized data bases containing the very latest medical information merely by inputting a desktop computer terminal connected electronically to all major world medical centers. When preliminary diagnosis indicates the need for specialized follow-up treatment, the physician, most likely using a computer, would have the capability of providing the patient with the most appropriate referral and would not hesitate to do so.

Unfortunately, this ideal of systematic medical practice does not yet exist. Many individuals, however, do have an established relationship with a physician, perhaps a specialist in family medicine, an internist, or a cardiologist. This physician offers the advantage of at least knowing something about the patient's medical history. Typically, men faced with problems of sexual dysfunction initially consult this physician. In the case of subscribers to health maintenance organizations (HMOs) or members of many group care health plans, there is usually no choice other than to contact a physician affiliated with the plan. This physician is often known as your "primary health care provider," or some similar designation.

What You Should Expect from Your Physician

It is unreasonable to expect your regular physician to be an authority on male sexual problems. On the other hand, you are entitled, at the very least, to the following when consulting your physician:

- ◆ Your problem should be received with understanding and concern. You should receive a full hearing, and under no circumstances should the importance of the problem be minimized. Your physician should make every effort to be reassuring, to put you at ease, and to help you in the difficult task of expressing your problem.

- ◆ A careful review should be made of your medical record, and your physician should give special attention to any history of high blood pressure, cardiovascular disease, diabetes, and other physical conditions and life-style problems, such as excessive alcohol intake, associated with male sexual dysfunction. Where indicated, the medical record should be supplemented with additional relevant tests.

◆ Your physician should review in detail the known adverse reactions of all medications that you are currently taking. If necessary, the physician should contact the indicated pharmaceutical manufacturers and professional colleagues for more complete information on possible side effects. Particular attention should be paid to drugs used in the treatment of high blood pressure. Where medically prudent, the physician should have no objection to prescribing alternative medications with possibly less serious side effects.

◆ If there is a reason to believe that your condition is due to prescription drugs or life-style problems, your physician should make appropriate recommendations and then carefully track the results over a reasonable period of time. If no change is noted in your problem, your physician should be prepared to carefully investigate the possibility that you have one or more of the known medical disorders associated with male sexual dysfunction.

◆ Should a condition that is strongly linked with sexual dysfunction be found, your physician should be prepared to immediately refer you to a urologist specializing in male sexual problems. Your physician may also suggest that you visit some other type of specialist, possibly an endocrinolgist, internist, or a cardiologist, when it is quite apparent that your sexual dysfunction difficulties are part of a broader medical problem requiring prompt treatment, such as a glandular disorder or a heart condition.

What Can Go Wrong

The following summarizes the experiences of Mort, a 59-year-old patient:

At age 35, the patient learned during a routine physical examination that he had moderately elevated blood pressure. His physician, an internist, prescribed an antihypertensive medication containing a diuretic and a tranquilizer. He did not warn the patient of the possible effect on sexual performance. Subsequently, the patient began to experience occasional episodes of impotence, which he told his doctor about during an office visit. In response, the physician stated that impotence was "almost always" psychological in origin, and thus terminated the discussion.

About five years later, the patient, now living overseas, experienced some pain while urinating and consulted a local urologist. The problem, traced to a prostate infection, was easily cured. In the course of treatment, the urologist warned of the possible adverse side effects of the patient's high blood pressure medication. The patient followed the urologist's advice, successfully controlled the hypertension problem through weight reduction, and discontinued the medication. The episodes of impotence became very infrequent.

Returning from overseas, the patient was thrown into a high-stress executive position. Given the all-too-frequent combination of stress and unavoidable business entertaining, the patient, in time was again significantly overweight. The patient, now age 50, had occasion to consult a physician regarding a gastrointestinal problem. The physician, a gastroenterologist, observing high blood pressure, insisted that the patient resume taking antihypertensives. This time, preparations of both the diuretic and beta blocker type were prescribed. Again, no warning was volunteered as to possible side effects. In a relatively short time, the patient was again experiencing impotence episodes. When the patient complained about this problem, he was told by the physician that impotence is a normal consequence of aging, and that he should not worry about it. The physician then changed the conversation to a discussion of the importance of an annual proctological examination. The patient's further attempts to bring up the subject of impotence proved futile.

Variations on the preceding story are heard almost daily by urologists specializing in male sexual dysfunction. Unfortunately, all too many physicians are still embarrassed by the subject or are fundamentally unsympathetic to the problem. Even when true concern exists, the physician may be poorly informed on the subject and too quick to attribute the patient's condition to psychological problems or aging.

Under no circumstances should you let your physician convince you that you are too old for sexual activities. In fact, if he or she attempts to do so, it is a good idea to get another physician, as such an opinion could indicate a practitioner who is uninformed on modern medical developments in general. It is worth noting that a 95-year-old patient was able to enjoy a successful sex life after having received a penile implant.

Some Specific Problems

Individuals seeking assistance may face special problems when dealing with group medical care providers. As mentioned, a subscriber to a health maintenance organization has no choice but to bring a problem of male sexual dysfunction initially to an HMO-designated physician. This situation can be expected to become increasingly common as the "managed care" approach to medical services grows in importance. Unfortunately, the chance exists that the designated physician could prove to be unsympathetic, unknowledge-able, or both, when it comes to male sexual dysfunction problems. Moreover, physicians in managed care programs are typically under pressure to minimize referrals to special-ists, as a means of controlling costs. Under such circum-stances, the subscriber must aggressively pursue the matter with the designated physician, or insist that another physi-cian be appointed under the plan. In extreme cases, there is little choice but to shift to an alternative medical program.

A problem can also exist in dealing with physicians in group medical practice. Group practice, in which perhaps a dozen physicians with different medical specialties join forces in a single corporate entity, and share physical facili-ties, accounting services, and so forth, is the fastest-growing segment of the medical profession. The growth of group practice is strongly stimulated by current underlying eco-nomic trends impacting on medical practice. In consulting a group practice, you should take into consideration the rea-sonable likelihood that an attempt will be made to refer all male sexual problems to group members. This could be a a problem when no member of the group has a strong capabil-ity in treating dysfunction.

Special problems also exist for individuals locked into medical programs based upon a specific employer. An ex-ample would be a member of the U.S. armed forces. Indi-viduals enrolled in such programs can face problems, both with respect to obtaining capable medical attention, and with respect to confidentiality. Preserving confidentiality could have important career implications. In some instances, there may be little choice but to seek specialized treatment on a private basis.

Finally, given the highly mobile U.S. population and other factors, many men do not have a regular physician. In such cases, it is reasonable to start directly with a urologist specializing in dysfunction. Various support groups and information services mentioned later in this chapter can prove useful in this connection.

THE ROLE OF THE UROLOGIST SPECIALIZING IN MALE DYSFUNCTION

Urologists are licensed physicians specializing in the treatment of problems of the urinary or urogenital tract. These include such problems as kidney, bladder, and urethra disorders. As such, a urologist may treat both men and women. In addition, urologists treat problems unique to men such as disorders of the prostate, penis, and testicles and male sexual dysfunction. Urologists are trained both as physicians and surgeons, and their practice may include performing the surgical procedures needed to treat urinary-genital problems. In recent years, the role of urologists in the treatment of "male trouble" has grown in importance. In many respects, urologists are assuming a role in the treatment of men parallel to that of gynecologists who treat "female trouble."

Until quite recently, the treatment by urologists of problems unique to men concentrated on such problems as prostate disorders, testicular disease, and conditions specific to the male urinary tract. As such, the treatment of male sexual dysfunction is quite new as a urology subspecialty. In view of the belated attention given to male sexual dysfunction, many excellent practicing urologists still do not enjoy strong capabilities in this area, including the necessary familiarity with diagnostic test procedures and treatment. This should be taken into consideration when seeking help. Appendix C includes the names of urologists who specialize in male sexual problems and are currently serving as regional medical advisors for the Impotence Institute of America.

What You Should Expect from Your Urologist

Unless your condition is especially complicated, a urologist specializing in male sexual dysfunction should be able to determine in two or three visits whether there are specific physical causes underlying your impotence or any other dysfunction problem. At least two visits are required before a positive treatment program can be recommended, because of the need to evaluate several important laboratory tests.

On the initial visit, you can expect the following:

◆ Being asked to complete a detailed medical history questionnaire (see sample in Appendix B)

◆ A lengthy detailed discussion with the urologist

◆ A detailed physical examination

◆ The taking of blood, urine, and prostate fluid samples for laboratory analysis

The initial discussion typically covers a review of dysfunction symptoms and your overall past medical history. You will be questioned as to the presence of nocturnal and morning erections and the frequency, duration, and quality of erections at other times. You will also be questioned as to your pattern of personal relationships, family- and job-related stress, and similar matters that may have possible psychological implications. Although this discussion will, by necessity, cover very sensitive areas, it will be to your advantage to respond as openly and completely as possible. Many urologists encourage the participation of the patient's sexual partner (if any) in the initial discussion, in view of the additional insight that may be provided.

The physical examination includes an inspection for abnormalities throughout the entire genital region, as well as observations and tests to provide evidence of any vascular, neurological, and hormonal difficulty. Inspection of the penis includes checking for scarring, Peyronie's disease, or any abnormal opening of the urethra. A digital rectal examination is made of the prostate, and a sample of prostate fluid is obtained for laboratory analysis. The testicles are examined as to size and any possible abnormality.

The vascular investigation includes the measurement of blood pressure of the penis and a comparison of this pressure with a blood pressure reading taken on the arm. The relationship of the two measurements is known as the penile-brachial index. Whenever penile blood pressure is found to be 65 percent or less of the normal arm blood pressure measurement, the possibility exists of insufficient blood supply to the penis. A "pulse volume recording" of how penile blood pressure varies over a period of time may be taken by placing a small blood pressure cuff around the penis and observing the results on a connected recording device. When the pulse volume recording reveals only minimal fluctuations in penile blood pressure over a period of time, the implications are some abnormality in the supply of arterial blood to the penis. A normal recording has a repetitive wave pattern characterized by significant "peaks" and "valleys."

Finally, the urologist will perform a series of tests to examine the key neurological reflexes in the genital and anal areas. These include observation of the bulbocavernosus reflex, as discussed in the previous chapter.

The subsequent laboratory analysis of body fluids is performed largely to determine the possibility of diabetes and hormonal problems, in particular abnormally low testosterone and abnormally high prolactin levels. A test to determine thyroid activity may also be run using the blood sample.

Tests the Urologist May Administer

Depending on the circumstances, your urologist may recommend that you take one or more of the following additional tests.

Arteriography

When there is reason to suspect that blockage of the arterial blood supply to the penis may underlie an impotence problem, it is possible to check, and even determine, the actual location of the abnormality with an arteriograph test. Arteriography, however, is usually recommended only in situations where there is a real indication of the need to perform arterial reconstructive surgery.

There are variations in test methods, but all involve the injection of a harmless solution into an upstream point in the arterial system. The injected solution moves downstream into the key blood vessels that supply the penis. As this takes place, X-ray photographs are taken at various angles of the pelvic area. The injected solution serves as a photographic contrast medium and permits the urologist examining the developed plates to determine the location and extent of any area of blockage. In some instances, the test may be performed with the penis in a drug-stimulated state of erection (see the discussion that follows).

Biothesiometry

Biothesiometry is a diagnostic technique that measures the sensitivity of the skin of the penis to mild vibrations. In performing the test, a small, mildly vibrating electromagnetic test probe, connected to a meter that measures vibration intensity, is placed at one point on the penis. While in place, the intensity of vibration is gradually increased until the point where movement is first detected by the patient. This intensity level, as indicated on the meter, is noted and the procedure is then repeated at several other locations on the penis.

The test provides a simple, and noninvasive, means of evaluating whether the sensory nerves of the penis are properly functioning. Often alcoholics and diabetics exhibit a low level of vibrational sensitivity when tested. The value of biothesiometry, however, is limited, as the procedure tells nothing about the proper functioning of other important nerves that have a role in causing erection.

Drug-stimulated Erection Testing

The use of the drugs in the treatment of impotence is discussed in Chapter 7. Drugs, however, are useful in diagnosis. In the test, a small quantity of a vasoactive drug is injected directly into the penis. In the past, papaverine was the drug most often used; however, in recent years prostaglandin E_1 has been increasingly preferred. When an erection does not take place shortly following injection, it indicates the possibility of a serious blockage in the arterial system blood supply to the penis or a leak in the downstream venous blood system, which could result in a failure to entrap or maintain blood in the corpora cavernosa when stimulus for an erection exists.

Corpora Cavernosagram

The taking of a corpora cavernosagram can be helpful in evaluating damage to the penis from Peyronie's disease, in detecting impotence possibly caused by leaking veins within the corpora cavernosa structure of the penis, or in treating a priapism episode. The test involves the injection of a photographic contrasting fluid into the penis, followed by a series of X rays. Measurements of blood pressure within the corpora cavernosa may be taken during the procedure. Some procedures may also involve stimulation of an erection and the taking of penile dimensions as the test proceeds.

Dynamic Infusion Cavernosometry

Dynamic infusion cavernosometry is an advanced test utilizing a drug-stimulated erection. In the procedure, a drug is injected into the penis with a resulting buildup of fluid pressure within the erectile tissues. Using suitable measuring instruments, the rate of drug infusion needed to maintain a sufficient level of pressure within the penis for erection can be determined and/or the time it takes for the pressure to return to normal levels.

The procedure can be used to evaluate the functioning of both the arterial system supplying blood to the penis and the venous system draining blood out of the penis. As in the case of arteriography, dynamic infusion cavernosometry is usually recommended only when there is evidence of a real need for reconstructive surgery.

Nerve Conduction Tests

Nerve conduction tests are used to determine the effectiveness of the nerve pathways employed for erection in the conducting of electrical impulses. These include the nerves in the penis, pelvic area, and spinal column. In the test procedure, electrodes are used to measure electrical characteristics associated with the bulbocavernosus reflex. An analogy exists with circuit testing procedures commonly used by electrical and electronic technicians in spotting circuit problems. When the bulbocavernosus reflex latency time is found to be abnormally long, there is an indication that some neurological problem may underlie impotence.

Nocturnal Penile Tumescence Monitoring

Nocturnal penile tumescence (NPT) monitoring, performed under medical direction, represents an advanced version of the simple home postage stamp test discussed in Chapter 5. NPT monitors vary in design and capabilities, depending upon the manufacturer. All monitors incorporate sensor mechanisms that are placed around the base and near the tip of the penis, permitting the continuous monitoring and recording of all changes that may occur in penile dimensions during rapid eye movement (REM) sleep. Examination of the hard copy produced by the monitor will reveal whether erectile activity has taken place. The result is considered positive when simultaneous expansion is noted at the base and tip of the penis. The newest, most sophisticated monitors also incorporate the capability to measure the rigidity of the penis, and thus provide a further indication of the potential ability to achieve normal vaginal penetration.

Depending upon the degree of accuracy required, NPT testing may be carried out at home, in the urologist's office, or in a hospital sleep laboratory. In sleep lab testing, more sophisticated equipment is used, and attendants are available to check on the equipment, to observe and grade penile rigidity, and sometimes to photograph erections. In some labs, the brain waves of patients are also monitored by electroencephalogram (EEG) devices, to determine the mode of sleep.

It is obvious that overnight testing in a sleep lab is an expensive proposition compared to office testing or testing at home using a portable NPT test. It is also far less convenient and more stressful to the patient. Such testing, however, can be required by some insurance carriers. Other carriers may accept testing done in physicians' offices or at home, or not require NPT testing at all. While NPT testing can provide useful results, many urologists do not routinely perform the tests, harboring reservations as to cost-effectiveness. Such urologists reason that adequate tools exist at less cost to the patient, including a simple test that can be performed overnight at home.

It is also important to be aware that the presence of an erection at night is not definite evidence of the ability to perform normal sexual activities. For example, a man subject to the steal syndrome, as discussed in the previous chapter, might very well be shown by the NPT test to have a favorable pattern of nighttime erections, but still experience difficulty in maintaining an erection during a period of intercourse. This should be kept in mind in dealing with an insurance company that relies heavily on NPT results in determining coverage of treatment. Such a company might be adverse to paying for a needed penile implant on the grounds that the NPT test would appear to indicate the absence of a physical problem.

Snap Gage Test

The relatively recent snap gage test represents a more sophisticated version of the simple postage stamp test for determining the presence of nocturnal erections that was discussed in the previous chapter. A specially designed rigid ring, containing three small plastic filaments, is placed around the penis before going to bed. The presence of nocturnal erections, and some indication of the degree of penile rigidity, is indicated by observing whether one or more of the plastic filaments are found to be broken upon getting up the next morning.

Dacomed Corporation, Minneapolis, Minnesota, a manufacturer of a snap gage device, emphasizes its value as an indicator of the degree of penile rigidity during nocturnal erections and its cost-effectiveness, as compared to traditional NPT testing. The same company also manufactures an ambulatory testing device that can be worn by a patient while active during the day, and which will measure and record the presence and degree of rigidity of any erections.

Ultrasonagraphy

Ultrasonography, often just referred to as "ultrasound," is a diagnostic technique in which sound waves are projected against some targeted part of the body. The sound waves that echo back from the target are converted to electrical energy and processed to form an image. Ultrasonography is based upon a principle of physics known as the Doppler effect and represents a medical version of sonar, a technique first used in naval warfare to detect the presence of submerged submarines.

When aimed at the penis, simple ultrasonography can be used to measure both arterial and venous blood flow. The procedure is noninvasive and painless. Duplex ultrasonography is a variation of drug-stimulated erection testing in which ultrasonogram images are taken before and after penile injection and, when compared, serve as an indication of the characteristics of blood flow.

Possible Tests of the Future

There is little doubt that many new and improved diagnostic tests will be making their appearance over the next few years. While recently in Russia, one of the authors witnessed a demonstration of an interesting device known as an acoustothermometer. This device, a by-product of aerospace technology, measures temperature gradients within the body with the use of a noninvasive ultrasonic probe. As abnormalities within the body are often associated with elevated temperatures, Russian scientists believed that an application may exist in the diagnosis of erectile dysfunction, as well as other medical problems.

When all necessary tests have been completed, your urologist will be in a position to provide a diagnosis of the problem and make specific recommendations. Possibilities could include drug or hormonal therapy, the surgical correction of vascular problems, or a penile implant. Referrals to other medical specialists may be appropriate when the impotence problem is found to be symptomatic of a medical condition such as diabetes. If no evidence of a physical cause can be found, referral to a sex therapist may be in order.

Most problems that arise with urologists who specialize in male sexual dysfunction usually involve unreasonable patient expectations. Brad, a 45-year-old recovered alcoholic, objected to the advice that a penile implant was the only effective solution to his problem. He was convinced that there was a miracle drug or operative procedure that could repair the permanent physical damage to his body caused by alcoholism. Ronald, age 50, was disappointed with the results of his implant. It had restored his sexual function, but it did not solve his other problem, a floundering personal relationship with his partner. Patients and partners, therefore, are advised to communicate fully their expectations to their urologist and to understand carefully the implications of the resulting advice.

THE ROLE OF PSYCHOTHERAPISTS AND SEX THERAPISTS

In cases where one or more physical causes of erectile dysfunction cannot be identified, referral to a psychotherapist or sex therapist is a logical step. Even in cases where impotence can be shown to be linked to physical factors, counseling will often prove very helpful, for both the man and his partner, to overcome the inevitable stresses associated with impotence and specific accompanying problems, such as performance anxiety.

Should you have a need for such treatment, it is very important to recognize that individuals calling themselves psychotherapists, sex therapists, or some similar term can differ widely as to education and training, surveillance of their professional activities by governmental or professional bodies, and treatment approaches. Individuals offering services related to male sexual dysfunction include psychiatrists, psychologists, social workers, religious counselors, hypnotists, and many others. Psychiatrists, of course, are licensed physicians with medical degrees. The educational credentials of others can range from no university degree to Ph.D.s.

Treatment approaches are also highly varied. In general, individuals calling themselves sex therapists tend to emphasize psychological conditioning techniques rooted in contemporary behavioral psychology theory. Psychological counselors, on the other hand, tend toward more conventional one-on-one or group therapy sessions. The former tend to attack the sexual problem directly, while the latter tend to explore broader aspects of the patient's background.

Many highly competent and reputable individuals are available for sex therapy or psychological counseling on sexual problems. The field, however, is subjective, and at this stage of knowledge, it is more an art than a science. Under these circumstances, it is not possible for governmental or professional regulation to fully protect the public from the ever-present possibility of quackery. In seeking treatment, therefore, it is wise to follow your urologist's referral. It is also advisable to contact a sex therapist or counselor affiliated with an accredited university or major medical center.

What You Should Expect from Your Psychotherapist or Sex Therapist

A discussion of the important specific treatment approaches used by psychotherapists and sex therapists appears in Chapter 9. The following summarizes what you are entitled to, in a general sense, when consulting such practitioners:

◆ Your therapist should request and review any information provided by your urologist or other relevant medical records.

◆ You should have ample opportunity to discuss the nature of your problem in detail at an extended initial meeting. At this interview, the therapist should not hesitate to provide information on professional credentials and qualifications relevant to treating problems similar to yours.

◆ You should be provided at the initial meeting, or soon thereafter, with a general appraisal of your problem and treatment prospects. A reputable therapist will not promise a miracle, but will offer an objective assessment of the probability of success based upon the information on hand regarding your individual circumstances and results observed in treating similar patients.

◆ Prior to the actual commencement of treatment, you should be fully informed as to the methods used in the treatment program. This should include specific information as to what will occur at treatment sessions, the length and frequency of sessions, and the degree of involvement, if any, of your partner. Anything unusual or possibly objectionable in the treatment program (for example, the possible use of female surrogates) should be made abundantly clear and agreed upon well in advance of the start of treatment. Any possible choices between alternative treatment approaches should also be made available at this time.

◆ While it is understood that it may be initially difficult to determine how long the treatment program will take, you should, nevertheless, be given a prelimi-

nary estimate of treatment duration and a full dis-
closure of associated costs.

◆   Throughout the entire program, the therapist should
    deal with you on a sympathetic and nonjudgmental
    basis. There should be a willingness to discuss your
    progress at any time during the program and, if
    indicated, to alter the treatment approach or termi-
    nate the program. There should also be a willingness
    to involve your urologist or other medical advisor in
    the program on a continuing and cooperative basis.

What Can Go Wrong

Despite the occasional, possibly lurid, horror story appearing in the popular media as to what may happen to individuals when they consult psychotherapists and sex therapists,
the most common problem is the expenditure of considerable sums of money for lengthy and ineffective treatment.
Robert had been unable to consummate his relationship with
his wife at any time over a period of seventeen years. Over
the period, both Robert and his wife had undergone intensive psychotherapy. Robert had been told that his problem
was due to repressed sexual feelings toward his mother.
When Robert turned up at a urologist's office, a simple test
of prolactin level revealed a reading of 180 units, as compared to the normal level of 11. Robert's problem, all along,
was caused by a pituitary tumor. The advanced stage of
Robert's tumor indicated that the problem causing impotence could have been detected years earlier.

The possibility of losing valuable time and money is
greatest when undertaking traditional psychoanalytical
treatment, which is by nature open ended, as compared to
the more structured approaches used in the sex therapy of
the Masters and Johnson type. It should be noted that most

proponents of traditional psychoanalysis do not attempt to hide the fact that treatment will be lengthy, sometimes arguing that it can take several years before sufficient rapport can be established to actually achieve results. Therefore, before you start any sex therapy, again first check for the possible existence of a physical problem.

Episodes of victimization by therapists, involving some form of sexual exploitation of the patient, do occur from time to time. Most such situations, however, are believed to involve female, rather than male, patients and, accordingly, are probably not often encountered by men being treated for sexual dysfunction.

SUPPORT GROUPS AND INFORMATION SERVICES

In recent years, a number of support and counseling groups concerned with male sexual dysfunction have been established. A list of such groups, and other organizations and individuals providing useful information on a national and sometimes international basis, is provided in Appendix C. Many local hospitals hold Impotents Anonymous meetings or meetings of similar organizations.

Impotents Anonymous (I.A.), probably the largest support group, dates to about 1981. The functions and activities of the organization have significant similarities with older support groups such as Alcoholics Anonymous. Local I.A. chapters are affiliated with the Impotence Institute of America, Inc., Washington, D.C., a nonprofit educational organization. Attendance at local I.A. chapter meetings is open, at no cost, to all individuals with an interest in the problem of impotence. Attendees have the option of placing their names on a chapter mailing list, which is kept strictly confidential.

Support groups, such as I.A., not only offer the opportunity for men and their partners to become better informed, but are also a unique outlet for individuals to share mutual problems. The following is the agenda of a fairly typical monthly meeting of the Atlanta, Georgia, I.A. chapter:

◆ Brief opening by the chapter coordinator

◆ VCR presentation of an educational film on impotence

◆ Lecture and slide presentation on impotence by a urologist specializing in male sexual dysfunction.

◆ Panel discussion—two couples relate their personal experiences

◆ Question-and-answer period, presided over by panel members and urologist

◆ Refreshments and informal discussion period

About 100 people attended this particular meeting, held in the cafeteria of a local hospital. Men made up slightly more than half the group. Most men were accompanied by their partners. The typical age of most present appeared to be in the 35 to 55 range, although many could have been considerably older or younger. About one out of ten in the group was African American. From casual conversation during the discussion period, it was evident that individuals present were from virtually all walks of life, including business executives, teachers, professional athletes, entertainers, and construction workers.

Despite the sensitive nature of the subject, the attendees, as a whole, participated actively in the discussions. Questions asked at the meeting ranged from defining the reasonable expectations of sexual performance to the fine details involved in the selection and use of penile implants. Those present showed little hesitation to tackle two really sensitive issues—the cost of treatment and what insurance companies will pay.

A typical meeting of Impotents Anonymous lasts about three hours. While there is never a charge for attendance, individuals can make a voluntary contribution to the refreshment fund. Meeting content varies, with the emphasis at many meetings on the psychological costs of impotence for both men and their partners.

Many attendees report that mere attendance at I.A. meetings can offer a distinct feeling of relief. This is partly the result of being made aware that you are not alone in your problem. The atmosphere of good humor and fellowship prevailing at meetings is undoubtedly a factor, as is the feeling of relief of actually initiating action to solve an all-consuming problem.

Active attendance at I.A. meetings is obviously not for everybody. The male and female lay coordinators of the Atlanta chapter have often provided useful information over the phone to both men and women who cannot or do not wish to attend meetings.

SUMMARY

This chapter has reviewed the basic options available to you if you seek help for a male sexual dysfunction problem. By learning as much as you can about your problem, asking the right questions (preferably in advance), and finding an informed physician, you can get the help you need.

TREATING IMPOTENCE WITH HORMONES AND DRUGS

For thousands of years, humankind has searched for a magical potion to cure impotence. Unfortunately, the results to date have been meager. At present, there are only a handful of hormones and drugs in the urologist's arsenal, testosterone, yohimbine, prostaglandin E1, papaverine, and few others. The pace of research is finally quickening, and it is expected that new and more effective drugs will become available over the next few years.

TESTOSTERONE

If you sample the blood testosterone levels of any large group of men of all ages and then plot, on a piece of graph paper,

137

the level of testosterone versus age for each man, the result is a confused collection of dots scattered all over the piece of paper. Looking closer, or better still, having a computer do the job for you, a pattern can be observed. Testosterone levels are negligible below the age of 10. Then the level rises steeply through approximately age 25. The rise continues, but at a much slower rate, to peak in the mid- to late thirties. Then it declines slowly through the remaining years.

The confused appearance of the pattern occurs because many men differ widely from the norm. Occasionally, a man at age 80 may have double the testosterone level of most men of his age. On occasion, a man at age 25 may have half the normal level for his age. The wide variations are the result of a number of factors: disease, excessive use of alcohol, hormonal therapy for prostate problems, physical injury, exposure to toxic substances, the malfunctioning of the hypothalamus and pituitary glands, or perhaps just the genes.

Phillip, a patient, age 42 could not understand his lack of sexual drive, low level of energy, and lack of muscular strength. His blood testosterone level turned out to be only 22, about the level of a 10-year-old boy. It should have been in excess of 500. Phillip was greatly helped by a testosterone supplementation program.

Before you conclude that testosterone is the cure for your problem, it is important to be aware of a few facts. Many men are able to perform very well despite abnormally low testosterone levels. Only about one quarter of all men with abnormally low testosterone levels and sexual performance problems will respond favorably to the treatment. In general, such men are also experiencing loss of libido. Testosterone supplementation does virtually nothing for men with normal levels. To make matters worse, excessive levels of testosterone supplementation can exacerbate benign prostate enlargement and prostate cancer. Remember, castration is not uncommon in treating men for prostate cancer. There is no evidence, however, that testosterone therapy triggers prostate cancer in men free of the disease.

As a result, testosterone supplementation should be undertaken only under continuing medical direction. Unfortunately, it is sometimes possible to obtain the hormone without prescription.

There are basically three ways to replace deficient testosterone in the body. The first is to take the hormone orally. Oral tablets on the market are in the methyltestosterone form. Taking the drug orally is convenient, but it is not recommended, due to problems in controlling dosage levels. Some of the problems that may occur with improper usage include, in addition to the possibility of worsening an existing prostate enlargement or prostate cancer condition, impaired liver function, kidney damage, and fluid retention.

A better way to raise the testosterone level is with intramuscular injections. This type of treatment starts with a series of trial injections in the urologist's office. The testosterone used is usually in the enanthate form; the dosage level initially used is in the 100- to 200-milligram range, depending upon one's weight and the degree of deficiency. If the treatment is found to improve sexual performance, the injections are repeated every two weeks. Often, in addition to an improvement in performance, increased body vigor and a more enthusiastic mental state are experienced.

With suitable instructions, testosterone injections can continue at home, with injections carried out either by the patient or by his partner. An alternative preferred by many patients is to have small, slow-release testosterone pellets implanted under the skin. The procedure is done in the urologist's office, takes about 15 minutes, and except for the quick injection of a local anesthetic, is painless. The pellets are usually implanted in the upper back, a few inches below the left or right shoulder. Some patients experience swelling for a few days, itching, and minor discomfort. It is not a good time for weight lifting. Antibiotics are taken during this period to avoid infection. A testosterone pellet implant may prove effective for a period of six months to one year.

At the present time, experimental work is underway on the possible use of skin patches containing testosterone. If successful, this will permit the slow release of testosterone from a small adhesive patch placed on the scrotum.

Long-range work is currently underway in connection with the hormonal chemical known as luteinizing hormone-releasing hormone (LHRH). This chemical is believed to play a key role in the mechanism by which the pituitary gland, located in the base of the brain, controls the production of testosterone in the testicles. This work may ultimately result in a convenient way to raise hormonal levels.

YOHIMBINE

Yohimbine, usually in hydrochloride or lactate form, is a chemical substance that has some benefit in the treatment of impotence. This drug was originally obtained from the dried bark of the corynanthe johimbe tree or closely related tree species found in various countries of central Africa and India. Yohimbine is also known as quebrachine, corynine, and aphrodine. The drug can now be produced commercially by chemical synthesis.

For hundreds of years, yohimbine was used in folk medicine as an aphrodisiac. In fact, it was one of the few aphrodisiacs with any real evidence of effectiveness. Early in the twentieth century, the drug was used on a limited basis by physicians in the treatment of impotence. In the mid-1940s, the drug was rediscovered and used essentially on an experimental basis. In many recent studies, yohimbine has been tested in a product that also contains methyltestosterone.

Yohimbine's aphrodisiac properties are believed to be due to the erotic effect the drug has on the brain and central nervous system. The drug's effectiveness in treating impotence, however, is believed to be mainly related to its action as an adrenergic blocker. In this capacity, the drug blocks certain portions of the sympathetic nervous system that have a role in inhibiting erection. Yohimbine also serves to promote an increased flow of blood to the penis.

In general, yohimbine has been used most successfully in the treatment of impotent men with diabetes. The scientifically manufactured drug is available in tablet form from urologists. Ground johimbe tree bark or yohimbine-containing lotions of questionable effectiveness, however, are sometimes available through health food stores and by mail order. Such products are often sold with claims that are very questionable and in bad taste. For example, a recent mail order solicitation for a "Yohimbe Erection Lotion" contained the statements, "Just let your lady rub this strawberry-flavored treat on your favorite muscle and watch your fortunes rise" and "it's a mouthful that she will come back for again and again." The cost for 4 fluid ounces of this essentially useless product is $8.50.

Yohimbine must be used cautiously, and always under medical supervision. The drug has been found to increase blood pressure and, on occasion, cause nervousness, headaches, dizziness, and nausea. In fact, yohimbine has been used for the treatment of men and women with abnormally low blood pressure levels.

It has been said that as many as one quarter of all men with erectile dysfunction can be significantly helped by yohimbine therapy, and more will experience some degree of improvement. The drug is typically prescribed during the initial trial period at a level of three tablets per day, although higher dosages are sometimes recommended. About a two-month initial trial is needed to determine the effectiveness of the treatment. When the treatment is found to be effective, it is generally necessary to continue to take the drug indefinitely.

PENILE INJECTION THERAPY

Papaverine is a drug that acts as a vasodilator and muscle relaxant. It is used in the treatment of certain types of heart disease and for arterial spasms occurring in the brain. In the early 1980s, it was demonstrated that a solution of the drug injected directly by hypodermic syringe in the corpora cavernosa region of the penis would initiate a firm and long-lasting erection. Subsequent investigation of this phenomenon has resulted in a workable treatment for impotence, a useful diagnostic tool, and a vast increase in the knowledge of the mechanics of erection that will pay off in future years.

Richard, a 72-year-old patient, had been unable to achieve a firm erection for several years. After testing, his problem was found to be vascular or neurological in nature. Shortly after an injection of papaverine, Richard experienced an impressive erection that lasted for approximately three hours. After further testing and proper instructions, Richard was able to enjoy frequent and successful sexual activity at home.

In recent years, there has been a shift in penile injection therapy away from papaverine toward the use of prostaglandin E_1 or a combination of various drugs that act as vasodilators. Prostaglandin E_1 is a member of a family of drugs known as the prostaglandins, natural biologically potent lipid acids found in the seminal vesicles tissue of man and other mammalians. In the past, the principal use of prostaglandin E_1 has been the treatment of congenital heart defects in children. More recently, the drug has played a role in the use of the French abortion drug RU 486. When used instead of papaverine in penile injection therapy, prostaglandin E_1 has been found to act rapidly, lose its effect in an optimum period of time, and be associated with a lower level of undesirable side effects. It is more costly, however, and, in the case of some men, may cause greater pain when injected into the penis.

Drug combinations that are being used in penile injection therapy include various mixtures of prostaglandin E_1 , papavarine, and another vasoactive drug, phentolamine. A hormonal substance known as vasoactive intestinal polypeptide (VIP) has also been used in some combinations. VIP is a smooth muscle relaxant that has been found to be naturally present at high levels in the penis. The substance, which may serve as a neurotransmitter during erection, appears to have little effect when injected alone, but seems to strengthen the effect when used in drug combinations. There have also been clinical studies of a drug known as Certine, a mixture of papaverine and five other vasoactive agents. A reason for increasing interest in drug combinations is the possibility that the combination embodies the best properties of each individual drug, but by minimizing the total amount of any drug used, the undesirable side effect of any particular drug is kept to a minimum.

An obvious problem in the use of penile injection therapy is the perfectly understandable horror of most men at the thought of sticking a needle into the penis. The fear, however, is far worse than the reality. The drug is injected at a 45-degree angle into a side of the penis at its base using a fine, small-gage needle the same as that used by diabetics.

The actual pain may be described as a slight pinch. After the first few times, almost all patients overcome their fear.

The use of penile injection therapy involves the determination of proper dosage. After the first trial injection, the dosage level is experimentally increased or decreased until a level is obtained that results in an erection lasting about 45 minutes. The patient is monitored very closely during the procedure, watching for the possibility of unwanted side effects.

Patients typically have little trouble in learning how to inject themselves at home in preparation for sexual activity. For home injection, one option is for the patient to obtain a supply of hypodermic syringes prefilled with the proper quantity of the drug. An alternative option is for the patient to fill empty syringes from a sterilized bottle containing a supply of the drug.

Although the use of penile injection may appear to be at odds with the fun and spontaneity of sexual relations, most men and their partners do not find this to be a deterrent. Many couples make a game of the procedure, turning it into an enjoyable experience.

Penile injection therapy must always be used with caution, and all instructions should be carefully observed. The procedure should not be used by any man who is taking any drug classed as a monoamine oxidase inhibitor (MAOI), due to the possibility of a dangerous drug interaction. MAOIs are sometimes prescribed in the treatment of high blood pressure or depression. Penile injection therapy is also precluded in the case of men with an overwhelming aversion to the concept or who, due to a lack of manual dexterity, poor eyesight, or an inability to follow directions, are incapable of safely performing the procedure.

Penile injection therapy has now been used for a sufficient period of time to demonstrate relative safety and the absence of serious side effects. An immediate problem can arise, however, when an erection fails to relax over a prolonged period, such as up to six hours. This condition resembles priapism, but is normally not true priapism. Prolonged erections are rare, especially when instructions are followed.

Men who use injection therapy are instructed to contact their urologists promptly whenever an erection lasts more than four to six hours. Under such circumstances, the urologist usually terminates the erection with an injection of a diluted saline solution containing adrenalin (epinephrine). The injection neutralizes the effect of the injected drug, with the result that the dilated vessels carrying blood into the penis constrict, thus impeding the passage of blood into the penis. The urologist may also find it necessary to draw some blood out of the penis.

Using penile injection therapy more than two times per week or at intervals of less than two days is not recommended, due to the possibility of scarring, as revealed by lumps and nodules in the penis. Too-frequent use can also result in bruising, itching, and bleeding. Long-term use may result in fibrosis or scarring of the penis, or possibly a curved erection. After a period of time, the particular drug being injected may gradually lose its effectiveness. In such circumstances, the patient may be helped by a shift to an alternate drug or drug combination.

Penile injection therapy provides a useful short-term solution for men who ultimately may elect to have a penile prosthesis installed but wish to avoid immediate surgery. Penile injection therapy has a success rate of about 70 percent, and it has been reported that in excess of 200,000 men are now employing the procedure. Although the drugs used in penile injection therapy all have the approval of the U.S. Food and Drug Administration (FDA) in connection with their traditional uses, penile injection therapy itself and the use of the indicated drugs in this particular medical application still does not enjoy specific approval. It should be noted, however, that when the FDA approves the sale of any drug for a given application, that drug may be used with caution in other applications. In general, penile injection therapy has advanced well beyond the point where it is considered just experimental in character, but it is still a procedure that can be employed only under close medical supervision.

OTHER DRUGS

Several other drugs are being used for the treatment of impotence, some on an experimental basis. As mentioned in Chapter 4, bromocriptine mesylate has been found to improve erections in men with high levels of the female hormone prolactin. This drug, sold in tablets and capsules under the brand name Parodel for the treatment of female infertility and Parkinson's disease, has been found to lower prolactin levels and improve erections even in men with pituitary tumors. Such tumors are associated with abnormal prolactin secretion into the bloodstream. When the underlying problem is a tumor, use of the drug does not substitute for direct treatment of the tumor itself.

Propylthiouracil thyroid inhibitor "Propacil" is a drug used for the treatment of hyperthyroidism. This condition is sometimes linked to the loss of libido and erection difficulties. Use of the drug is often effective in improving both the thyroid and erection problem for many male patients.

Two drugs, whose usage been linked to undesired episodes of priapism, have been found, when used at proper dosage levels, to improve erectile dysfunction. The first is trazodone, a drug sold under the trade name Desyrel largely for the treatment of severe depression. When many male patients taking trazodone were found to experience priapism, the drug attracted interest as a possible impotence treatment. The drug, which is now being used sometimes in combination with yohimbine, has helped some patients and does not appear to affect the mental state of men not subject to severe depression. A second drug, levodopa, used largely in the treatment of Parkinson's disease, has also been linked to priapism. Encouraging results have been reported when the drug has been used as an experimental impotence treatment.

Some other drugs that have been investigated include pentoxifylline, oxytocin, and naloxone. Pentoxifylline, sold under the trade name Trental, is a drug used in the treatment of arterial disease. The drug appears to work by improving blood fluidity rather than as a vasodilator. Preliminary results on the use of this drug for the treatment of impotence are encouraging. Oxytocin is a drug used to induce labor in pregnant women. Naloxone is prescribed for the treatment of narcotic depression, resulting from the use of opium derivatives such as heroin. Preliminary studies reveal that both oxytocin and naloxone have a positive effect on erectile function.

The possibility that minoxidil may help to promote erection is an interesting story. This drug, which acts as a smooth muscle relaxant, was originally marketed under the Loniten trade name by The Upjohn Company, Kalamazoo, Michigan, as a high blood pressure medication. When it was found that many patients, both men and women, taking the drug were experiencing significant hair growth as an unexpected side effect, an extensive research effort was undertaken to develop a cure for baldness. This effort proved successful, with the company now marketing an FDA baldness remedy sold under the Rogaine brand name.

Rogaine is a topical solution of minoxidil that is applied directly to the scalp. As the effect is localized, there are minimal side effects, as compared to Lonitin, which is taken internally. Recently, it has been reported in some studies that topical solutions of minoxidil when applied to the glans penis (head of the penis) will promote erection. As the effect is again localized, presumably there should be minimal side effects.

With the recent discovery of the possible role of nitric oxide in the erectile process, the race has been been on to develop systems that will increase nitric oxide levels within the corpora cavernosa. One approach has been transcutaneous nitroglycerine therapy, the application of nitroglycerine to the surface of the penis in either the form of a patch or topical lotion. Nitroglycerine, a chemical probably best known for its use as a potent explosive, has been used for many years for the treatment of the painful heart condition known as angina pectoris. Nitroglycerine-containing patches applied to the chest have been found to be effective in relieving this condition.

To date, the use of nitroglycerine patches in the treatment of impotence has not been found to be overly encouraging, although work on this and related approaches is continuing. The principal problem appears to be the failure of sufficient quantities of the drug to penetrate through the tough barrier of the tunica albuginea into the corpora cavernosa. In the case of chest patches, the chemical, in contrast, appears to be able to easily reach the areas where it is needed. Another problem with use of nitroglycerine is that the drug, when applied to the penis, can penetrate through the vagina of the female partner and cause side effects, such as headache. Use of a condom, however, will eliminate this possibility.

Work is also known to be underway on the possible use of a suppository containing a gel with one or more drugs that promote erection. The suppository would be inserted directly into the urethra. Insertion should not be painful or difficult as demonstrated by the inclusion of medicated salves intended for urethral insertion that were a standard item in the "pro kits" distributed in the past to American servicemen as a means of protecting against sexually transmitted disease. No clinical information is yet to be available as to the effectiveness of the suppository approach.

SUMMARY

An increasing number of important drugs for treating impotence are finally becoming available that demonstrate real results in many patients. All available drugs, however, must be used with care and under a urologist's supervision. Penile injection therapy, which only dates to the decade of the 1980s, is now a well-accepted approach to the treatment of erectile dysfunction. Use of penile injection therapy has also made a major contribution to an understanding of the causes and treatment of erectile failure. No form of drug treatment available to date, including penile injection therapy, has proven to be a universal cure-all, but help has been provided to many patients. There is little doubt that vastly improved treatments involving drugs will be making their appearance in the very near future.

TREATING IMPOTENCE:

USE OF PENILE IMPLANTS, VASCULAR SURGERY, AND EXTERNAL VACUUM DEVICES

The following letter was received from a patient a few weeks after he had a penile implant:

> *Dear Doc,*
> *I have to be careful not to sleep on my stomach any more, inasmuch as I might puncture my water mattress.*
> *You sure do good work, and now due to your good work, I'm doing pretty good work.*

151

This chapter deals with the various techniques, other than the use of hormones and drugs, that are now available for the treatment of impotence. Much of this chapter deals with prostheses that are surgically implanted in the penis. By definition, a prosthesis is any device that replaces or substitutes for a missing or nonworking body part. A dental plate is a common example of a prostheses. A penile prosthesis is commonly referred to as a penile implant, or simply an implant.

Several surgical procedures being used to correct venous or arterial vascular problems linked to impotence are also discussed in this chapter. At present, there is little that can be done to deal surgically with neurological defects that result in impotence, although work in the repair of neurological damage, in general, is underway and is very promising.

The use of prostheses was pioneered in the United States, and has turned out to be the most common solution to date involving surgery among Americans. Vascular surgery for impotence was largely pioneered in Europe, and is still most common with Europeans. In time, it is reasonable to expect that practice throughout the world will include the appropriate use of both surgical approaches.

Finally, this chapter also includes a discussion of external vacuum devices designed to provide an erection. Such devices represent a nonsurgical approach to the treatment of erectile dysfunction.

PENILE IMPLANTS

As noted in Chapter 2, penile implants have become available on a regular basis only since the 1970s. Since then, the estimated total number of such devices inserted in patients in the United States is about 200,000. In excess of 25 percent of all implants have been, according to one report, in men with erectile dysfunction resulting from diabetes. The second largest group, in excess of 15 percent, have been in men experiencing impotence following radical pelvic surgery for the treatment of prostate tumors or bladder or colon problems. Impotence due to vascular defects or physical injury accounts for about 10 percent each of all implants. The remaining number of implants were widely distributed among men subject to impotence due to other problems.

Regarding the factor of age, the largest number of implants, about 31 percent, has been reported to be in men in the 50- to 59-year-old age group. Men age 60 to 69 account for about 26 percent, and the 40 to 49 age group accounts for about 21 percent. Many men age 70 and older, however, have had implants, including quite a few men age 80 and older. Men with implants can father children. This was the case with a 29-year-old patient who had never before been able to have successful sexual intercourse.

The overall success rate for penile implants among all American men has been reported to be about 90 percent. In our practice, we have installed over 1,000 implants during the past fourteen years. The revision rate following treatment has only been in the 3 to 5 percent range. Only 1 percent of all patients experienced infection as a postoperative complication.

Several American companies are now manufacturing prostheses for a growing market, both in the United States and overseas. The rapid acceptance of implants reflects the fact that such devices represent a very pragmatic solution to the impotence problem.

Types of Implants

At present, four basic types of implants are available: the semirigid malleable prosthesis, the simple self-contained inflatable prosthesis, and the more complex two- and three-piece inflatable protheses. Photographs of products in each category are shown on the following pages. The positioning of the inflatable implant within the penis and the lower body cavity is also shown in an accompanying drawing. A description of the types of implants and their respective advantages and disadvantages follows.

Semirigid Malleable Implant

Semirigid malleable implants, as shown in Figures 8-1 and 8-2, are relatively simple devices and the first implants to be used on a large scale. Many different products of this nature have been developed by different manufacturers. Most semirigid malleable implants incorporate rods made of an inert plastic material. Some also incorporate a flexible metal of stainless steel or silver wire, both highly inert metals. The semirigid malleable implant manufactured by American Medical Systems, Minneapolis, Minnesota, shown in Figure 8-1, incorporates two rods made of silicone, an inert elastomeric substance, along with a stainless steel core. The device manufactured by the Dacomed Corporation, Minneapolis, Minnesota, shown in Figure 8-2, is made of ultrahigh-molecular-weight polyethylene and is based on a design that incorporates a series of positionable internal plastic segments, along with a stainless steel core.

When a semirigid malleable implant is surgically placed in the penis, a permanent erection results. The penis and implant can, however, be bent down close to the body so that it will not be noticed under most clothing. When intercourse is desired, the penis is merely straightened. This is easily accomplished with just one or two fingers. The Dacomed Corporation claims that its device provides superior concealability given its special interior design.

The principal advantage of a semirigid device is cost, both for the device itself and for implantation. The surgical

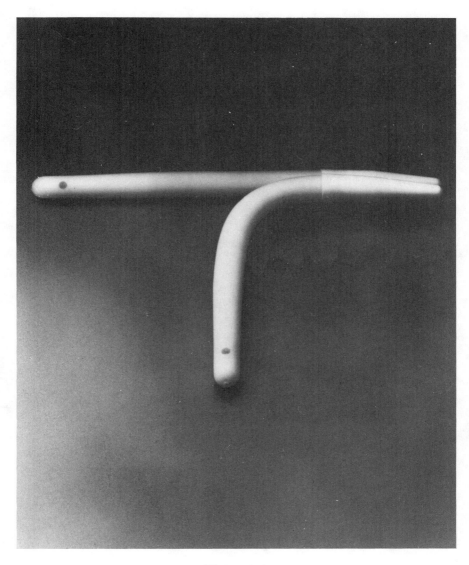

Figure 8-1
Semirigid Malleable Implant
Courtesy of American Medical Systems
Photograph by Mike Schenk

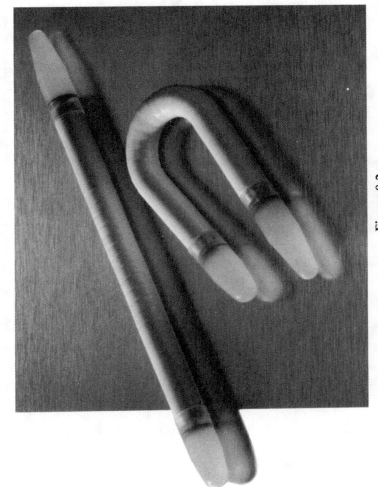

Figure 8-2
Semirigid Malleable Implant
Courtesy of The Dacoma Corporation

procedure is simpler than with other types and adapts to implantation on an outpatient basis. Another advantage is that there is no need for pumping prior to intercourse or deflating afterward, both of which might detract from the enjoyment of the situation in some men and their partners.

The principal disadvantage is the permanent erection. This could be a problem to a man when wearing a tight bathing suit or aerobic outfit or when changing clothes in a public locker room such as in a health club or gymnasium. The erection, while generally adequate, is not characterized by an increase in the length or girth of the penis. There is also a possibility of springback in which the implant straightens out on its own from the position in which the penis has best concealment. Dacomed claims to have superior properties in this respect. Finally, there is the remote possibility of perforation of the penis, although, in general, the need for possible reoperation in the case of a semirigid malleable implant is lower than with inflatable devices.

Simple Self-Contained Inflatable Implant

The simple self-contained inflatable implant made by American Medical Systems, as shown in Figure 8-3, consists of two cylinders that are inserted entirely within the penis. Each cylinder contains an inert hydraulic fluid. When an erection is desired, it is easily obtained by squeezing the end of each rod located near the front of the penis. The erection can be easily eliminated by bending the penis at its base or by pressing the relief valves within the mechanism. The self-contained inflatable implant made its appearance in 1984.

The self-contained inflatable implant offers the advantage of an erection that can be controlled at will. As a consequence, there is no concealment problem. It is more expensive than the semirigid type, but less expensive than

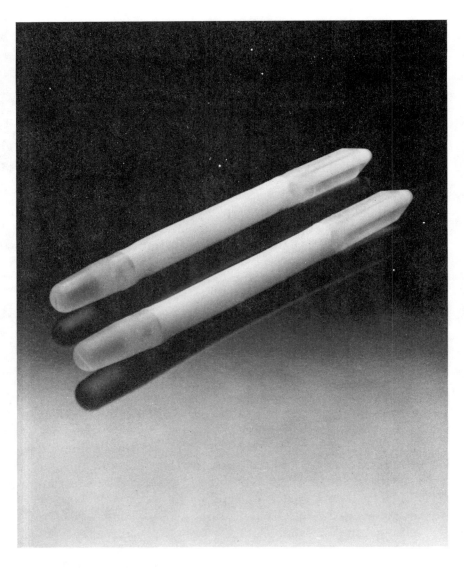

Figure 8-3
Simple, Self-Contained Inflatable Implant
Courtesy of American Medical Systems
Photograph by Mike Schenk

158

the more complex three-piece inflatable device. The surgical procedure required is relatively simple, although somewhat more complicated than the semirigid malleable implant. One possible disadvantage is that it does not provide a particularly full erection, compared to other inflatable implants, as there is no increase in the length or girth of the penis. However, this is rarely found to be a problem. Another disadvantage is that at times the device may deactivate on its own during intercourse.

Two-Piece Inflatable Implant

The two-piece inflatable implant is a relatively new development dating to about 1988. The implant contains two basic elements, two parallel hollow cylinders that are surgically placed in the penis and a bulb-shaped chamber containing both a reservoir for the hydraulic fluid and a pump which is placed within the scrotum. The two-piece inflatable implant made by the Mentor Corporation, Santa Barbara, California, is shown in Figure 8-4. The Mentor device is fabricated from polyurethane, a tough plastic material that resists distention.

A major advantage of the two-piece inflatable implant is that it provides a more naturally appearing erection than is the case with either the semirigid malleable and simple self-contained inflatable implant types. Another important advantage is that the two-piece inflatable device does not necessitate the surgical placement of a hydraulic reservoir in the lower abdominal cavity, as is the case with the three-piece inflatable implant, as discussed next. Such placement can be a problem in men who have previously experienced abdominal surgery for various conditions, including treatment of prostate tumors and even hernias. The major disadvantages, as compared to the semirigid malleable and simple self-contained inflatable type, are that surgical insertion is more

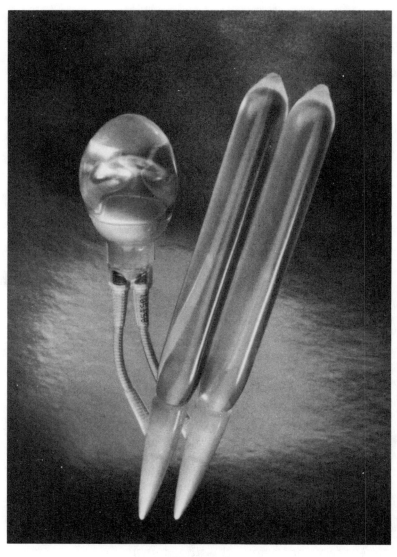

Figure 8-4
Two-Piece Inflatable Implant
Courtesy of Mentor Corporation

complicated and there are more parts to possibly malfunction.

Three Piece Inflatable Implant

The three-piece inflatable implant manufactured by American Medical Systems, as shown in Figure 8-5, has been available since the mid-1970s. Advanced versions of this device offer the best erection possible, including increased erect penile length and girth. Three-piece inflatable implants contain three basic elements. The first element consists of two parallel hollow cylinders that are placed within the penis. The second element is a pump and valve mechanism that is placed within the scrotum, close to the testicles. The third is a spherical reservoir containing hydraulic fluid that is placed inside the lower abdomen. Three tubes, entirely inside the body, connect the reservoir to the pump and the pump to each cylinder. The hydraulic fluid used is a safe mixture of sterile salt water and diluted X-ray contrast material. The pump can be placed in either the right or left side of the scrotum, depending on personal preference.

This device is easily inflated by squeezing the pumping mechanism inside the scrotum a number of times, which results in fluid moving into the cylinders. When the erection is no longer desired, it is easily deactivated by compressing the release valve on the side of the pump. The fluid then returns to the reservoir and the erection disappears.

The three-piece inflatable implant offers the advantages of maximum control and the most authentic-appearing erection in terms of added penis length and increased girth. The disadvantages are higher cost and the more involved surgical procedure that is needed. Also, since the device is more complex, there is a greater possibility of malfunction. Despite these disadvantages, however, the majority of men in the past have opted for the more complex inflatable device.

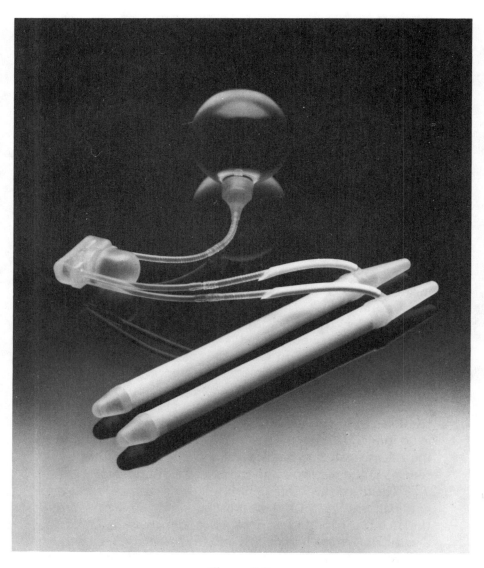

Figure 8-5
Three-Piece Inflatable Implant
Courtesy of American Medical Systems
Photograph by Mike Schenk

Continuing product improvement, including design changes and the use of superior materials, has resulted in less time needed in surgery and greatly reduced occurrence of malfunction for all four basic types of implants. There is little doubt that this trend will continue.

Implant Surgery

Both the semirigid and the simple self-contained inflatable prostheses are inserted surgically through an opening made by the surgeon in the penis. The procedure is relatively simple and may not require a hospital stay.

The implantation of an inflatable prothesis of the nonself-contained type is the most complicated procedure and is usually performed in a hospital setting. A skilled urologist, however, can perform the procedure in as little as 30 minutes and, in many instances, on an outpatient basis. Procedures are also becoming quicker and easier as urologists specializing in the area gain more experience. Depending on the preferred procedure, the device is inserted through a small opening below the base of the penis or in the lower abdominal cavity. The three major elements of the device are then placed in the desired positions, as shown in Figure 8-6.

In the surgical procedure, the patient does not have to have general anesthesia, as the use of a spinal or local type anesthesia is possible. Some patients, of course, may prefer full anesthesia. Patients typically are hospitalized for one to three days. Most patients are back to work in one week. Full recovery may take up to four weeks, and sexual intercourse should be possible by the fourth to sixth week. Patients receive careful instructions for the recovery period.

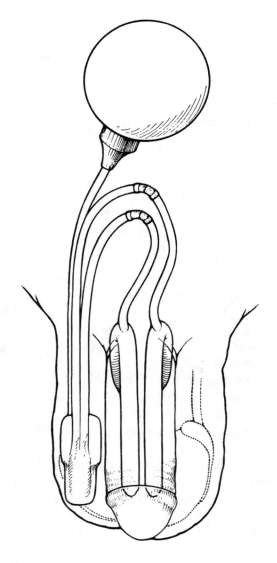

Figure 8-6
Drawing Showing Location of Inflatable Implant Within the Body
Courtesy of American Medical Systems
Photograph by Mike Schenk

164

Results

Based on information provided by the author's patients, favorable results are reported in excess of 90 percent of the cases. There is no evidence that the implant interferes with normal sexual intercourse, sexual desire, penile sensation, or fertility. Patients who were able to achieve orgasm or ejaculate before receiving the implant are fully capable of doing so afterward. Insertion of an implant, however, will permanently alter the erectile tissues of the penis so that a man receiving an implant will be dependent upon having an implant to engage in future sexual intercourse.

As mentioned previously, men with adequate sperm production are perfectly capable of fathering children after having received an implant. This, of course, obviously does not apply in the case of men who have had vasectomies.

Some typical results and comments obtained from our continuing mail survey of former patients are revealing. These include the following:

> *Are you satisfied with how hard your penis is when it is in the "up" position?*

Almost all former patients check the "yes" answer. A patient who qualified a positive response with the word "almost" nevertheless indicated strong general satisfaction in subsequent questions.

> *Are you satisfied with how your penis looks in the "down" position?*

The answers to this question are almost unanimously positive. Comments range from "very" to "it is A-okay" to "mighty proud."

Overall, are you happier since your penile implant?

Again the response is almost always "yes." Some comments include "much," "very," and "definitely." One especially articulate former patient commented as follows: "Absolutely. It's like getting the keys to the candy store."

Knowing what you know now, would you still have decided to have an implant?

The response to this question is strongly positive. Comments range from a simple "damn right" to the following: "I'm only sorry I did not know of this technique sooner! I feel and believe I act younger–all impotent men should have this!"

If such a thing were possible, is there anything you would change about your prosthesis?

Almost all responses to this final question were negative. An articulate patient added the comments, "I am completely happy with it, and so is my wife. I don't know how it could be improved." According to another patient, "It's the only operation I've ever enjoyed." A third patient added: "I should have had it done ten years ago."

The Implant Decision

The decision to have an implant should never be taken lightly. It is a decision that involves a major medical procedure and financial expense, as well as the patient's partner and life-style. Any man considering an implant should be well informed on the subject and review all aspects of the matter with his urologist and his partner. Talking to men who have had implants, and their partners, can also be very useful. Such people can be contacted through impotence support groups. Some factors that will influence the implant decision are illustrated by the following examples.

Case 1: A Man with No Other Choice

Larry, a 60-year-old truck driver, very much desired to have sexual relations with his partner, but this had not been possible for the past five years. Unfortunately, his impotence was due to irreversible physical damage resulting from alcoholism. Fortunately, he had stopped drinking, but it was too late to restore function. An attempt to use penile injection therapy proved unsuccessful, as did other alternatives. For Larry to ever again enjoy normal sexual activity, an implant was the only option.

Case 2: A Man with Limited Choice

Walter, a retired 68-year-old corporate executive, had been experiencing impotence for about two years. He was in excellent health, and medical examinations revealed no physical condition that could be connected to impotence. A good possibility existed that Walter's problem was psychological in nature, possibly associated with life-style changes necessitated by retirement. Walter chose an implant over some form of psychological or sex therapy. A very private and strong-minded person, Walter objected to any form of treatment that would involve the exposure of his feelings. He reasoned, probably correctly, that given his general attitudes, he would be a very poor candidate for successful treatment of a psychological nature. In Walter's words, "At my age, anything other than an implant would be a waste of time and money."

Case 3: A Man with a Possibly Viable Alternative

Charles, a 35-year-old university professor, had been experiencing impotence symptoms for about six months. When examined, he was in generally good health, although he had been drinking and smoking more than usual since the impotence problem began. No definite physical problem linked to impotence could be detected by examination.

Charles was anxious to have an implant. He was encouraged, however, to first undertake a program of sex therapy and to defer a possible implant until the results of such treatment became apparent. The results were favorable and an implant was not found to be necessary.

Some Common Concerns About Penile Implants

Concern 1: I would like an implant, but I am frankly worried about the operation. Is it safe? What will happen? Will it be painful? Will anybody find out?

All surgical procedures have some degree of risk, but there is little to be concerned about when the installation of a penile implant is performed by a urologist specializing in the area. Even in a very simple operation, such as having your tonsils removed, occasionally a patient will have an adverse reaction to the anesthesia. Local infection is also a possibility, and does occur in roughly 1 to 2 percent of the cases. Bleeding and retention of urine sometimes occurs on a temporary basis following the operation. Penile scarring can occasionally occur.

The most involved of the procedures requires being admitted to the hospital as an inpatient. In this case, the patient is admitted to the hospital on the morning of the surgery or perhaps the night before. Routine tests and a preoperative examination are performed. The patient will be visited by an anesthesiologist, and anesthesia options will be fully discussed. Usually, the patient will receive one or more injections of intravenous antibiotics prior to the operation and, when desired, an injection of a suitable tranquilizer.

The operation itself is not especially painful, as it is done with appropriate anesthesia. The patient is usually on his feet and getting around easily shortly after the operation. The patient is also usually able to resume eating on the day of surgery. Some mild localized discomfort is common during the recovery period, associated with the healing incision. The pain and discomfort gradually diminish and, in any event, can be controlled with suitable medication. When healing is complete and pain fully disappears, the patient is no longer aware of the presence of the implant. The situation is much the same as wearing a wristwatch—it is something that you are not aware of until you want to use it.

Privacy is a very real and justifiable concern of most men. The time spent in the hospital, and the overall recovery period, are sufficiently short so that the entire matter can take place during a brief vacation period. This was Donald's approach. The 50-year-old business executive checked into the hospital over the Christmas holidays. He commented that he was giving a Christmas present to himself. The only people who ever knew he was there were the involved medical personnel, the insurance company, and his partner.

Concern 2: Will my partner find the implant somehow objectionable?

No statistical survey of partners has ever been conducted that we are aware of that would answer this question conclusively. There is, however, considerable case evidence, based on interviews with partners and comments made at meetings of impotence support groups, that the entire sexual process feels natural and fully satisfactory. Some female partners comment that with the implant the pressure to perform is removed, allowing both partners to find the sexual experience more enjoyable than ever before.

Actually there is very little obvious evidence of the existence of an implant. In rare instances, some men with implants have reported that partners who have not been made aware of the existence of the implant have not sus-pected its presence.

Concern 3: Is it "natural"?

Walter, a patient with vascular insufficiency, was wor-ried that a penile implant is "just not natural." Walter ex-plained that he would only buy "natural" vitamins and other products at a health food store. He would wear only clothes made of wool and cotton, never synthetics. He proudly advised that he would never use pesticides or synthetic fertilizers on the tomato plants he grew each year. Walter, however, also wore glasses, had several dental crowns, and had been inoculated against all the common contagious dis-eases.

A penile implant, of course, is not natural, in much the same sense that riding in an automobile or flying in an airplane is not natural. It does, however, allow a man to engage in normal sexual activity that feels natural in all respects. Walter's actual problem was that he had been con-ditioned to believe that a real man never has trouble achiev-ing a supererogation. It never occurred to Walter that if sex is only to be performed under perfectly natural conditions, all forms of contraception would be automatically ruled out, including abstinence from sex during the female partner's fertile periods. After a successful implant, Walter was the first to admit he had been wrong.

Concern 4: I am a very active person. Will the presence of an implant cause a problem?

Men with implants include heavy construction workers and at least one professional wrestler, and they have no difficulty in engaging in vigorous sports, including running, tennis, weight lifting, and bicycle riding. There is, of course, the "locker room problem" associated with the semirigid prosthesis, as discussed previously.

Few sports place as much physical stress on the groin area as do horseback riding and polo. Yet one former implant patient continues to play a vigorous game of polo and reports no unfavorable consequences.

Concern 5: I feel guilty about the expense.

Money is always a consideration. As seen in Chapter 11, the total expense after insurance is often not unreasonable. The enjoyment of normal sexual activity is not a personal indulgence, but an essential part of life for most adults in our society. The cost of treatment is actually less than the emotional cost of nontreatment.

Concern 6: I feel guilty about not solving the emotional problems causing my condition.

This statement implies a belief that impotence is always caused by psychological factors. This, as you now know, is definitely not the case. Some sex therapists will hint that it is a sign of weakness to decide on an implant, rather than embark on a program of sex therapy, when the underlying problem appears to be entirely psychological. In the case of older men, with obviously limited life expectancy, the choice of an implant can be very logical and certainly nothing to feel guilty about.

Concern 7: Impotence and incontinence are both often a result of prostate surgery. Is it possible to install a penile implant and an artificial urinary sphincter in a patient subject to both problems?

Damage to the pubococcygeus muscles during prostate surgery frequently results in incontinence. An artificial urinary sphincter is a prosthesis designed to exert pressure on the urethra in the same area as the damaged natural sphincter in order to stop involuntary voiding. The device employs a hydraulic system similar to that used in a penile implant. Adequate space exists within the male body for the installation of both an artificial urinary sphincter and a penile implant, and this has been accomplished and proven satisfactory in many patients.

Concern 8: Will problems develop using the implant?

The chemically inert materials used in available prostheses have been carefully selected to avoid health hazards. Similar materials are regularly placed inside the body in connection with other forms of medical treatment without problems developing.

There is, as has been previously discussed, a possibility of the implanted prosthesis malfunctioning, which will necessitate surgical removal and replacement. This, as noted, is becoming far less common, due to continuing improvements in technology.

Some patients feel that the possibility of a malfunctioning prosthesis is a small price to pay for regained sexual vigor. For example, Bernie had been very pleased with his implant, but, to his considerable regret, the device stopped working after five months. X-ray examination revealed that there was a rupture in the cylinder, and the hydraulic fluid had escaped. Without hesitation, Bernie decided on a prompt replacement, which has provided excellent service ever since. Bernie views the matter philosophically, advising that he has twice replaced defective fuel pumps in an expensive late-model automobile. Implant manufacturers, incidentally, usually offer lifetime warranties on their products. The other costs of replacement, such as surgery, however, do have to be accounted for.

A second problem is that a relatively small number of men have difficulty adjusting to the idea that an implanted device is substituting for what they think should be a natural consequence of their manhood. At times, such men become morbidly preoccupied with the presence of the implant. This problem can be avoided if the urologist carefully screens patients before the operation. In many instances, this type of problem is due to unrealistic expectations as to how the implant will change the man's life.

Concern 9: Many penile implants use silicone plastic in their construction. Isn't there currently very serious concern about the use of silicones in female breast implants?

It is very true that concern does exist as to the use of silicone materials in breast implants; however, the situation is in no way comparable to that in penile implants. The typical breast implant has consisted of a pad with a flexible silicone plastic skin filled with a semiliquid silicone gel. This type results in a natural feeling, enlarged breast. The problems reported in women with defective breast implants have been associated with the escape of silicone gel material rather than the silicone plastic skin.

In the case of a penile implant, saline is employed as the fluid, not silicone gel. Saline is merely a solution of common table salt, sodium chloride. Saline is regularly injected into the body in many medical procedures, and blood, in effect, is essentially saline, plus some other substances. Should any saline escape from a penile implant, it would be harmlessly absorbed by the body. Such a situation, of course, might necessitate the replacement of the implant.

Concern 10: Are there medical conditions that would serve to preclude the use of an implant?

The number of conditions is relatively small. An implant would not make sense in a man with a serious medical illness and unable to withstand the normally minor stress of the surgical procedure. It may also not be possible to install an implant in a man with very severe penile scarring. The operation would also not be performed in the case of a man while subject to an active urinary infection or some similar difficulty.

VASCULAR SURGERY

Vascular surgery for impotence falls into two categories: procedures involving the venous system (which drains blood out of the penis) and procedures involving the arterial system (which supplies blood to the penis). Both approaches show promise, although there is a considerable amount of work, in general, that has to be done before vascular surgery becomes a major solution for the impotence problem. Most work in the field has taken place only during the past fifteen years.

Much of what is known regarding surgical procedures to correct abnormal drainage of blood from the penis has been learned as a result of treatment to correct the consequences of priapism. In treating an emergency priapism episode, the temporary drainage channel made by the physician to draw off blood may fail to heal properly, and persistent blood leakage causing impotence may be the unfortunate result. The procedure to treat this condition is not difficult and can be performed under local anesthesia. In the operation, the surgeon makes an incision near the front of the penis and cuts through to the damaged area that has been previously located by a corpora cavernosagram. The open channel is then sutured, resulting in the elimination of the leak.

The problem becomes more complicated when the patient has not experienced priapism, but a drainage problem is evident. A major problem in these cases is accurately pinpointing the open channel or channels responsible for the problem. When points of leakage can be properly identified from a corpora cavernosagram and a sufficient number of leaks corrected, the repair can be successful in many patients.

This was the case with Wayne, age 65, who had originally been scheduled for a penile implant. A second opinion revealed a simple leakage problem. A successful repair was achieved with a 15-minute surgical procedure.

Revascularization surgery to correct most arterial problems represents a major medical procedure, and is still at an early stage of development. One approach has been attempting to bypass the area where the critical arteries are blocked or are too narrow to permit adequate flow of blood to the penis. The bypass approach would be potentially most useful in treating impotence caused by arteriosclerosis. Unfortunately, this approach has not proven, to date, highly successful. One of the problems has been that just installing a bypass in one critical area will not eliminate the effect of arterial disease in the many small vessels supplying the penis. It should also be noted that bypasses installed in coronary arterial bypass surgery have been found to often close spontaneously within a period of ten years. This has led to a certain degree of current concern as to the effectiveness of coronary bypasses in the treatment of heart disease. The situation with regard to penile arterial bypasses is somewhat more discouraging: closure can take place in as few as six months.

Greater success has been achieved in the surgical removal of lesions impeding blood flow. Such lesions are usually caused by physical injury and represent a frequent cause of impotence in younger men.

In general, vascular surgery is recommended only for highly selected patients. Only an estimated 5 percent of all men with erectile dysfunction are considered good candidates for the procedures available at the present time. A very specialized person is needed to perform the surgery, not the typical general urologist. Complications are possible, including infection, penile scarring, and painful erections. There is also evidence of a high rate of recurrence of impotence after surgery. Fortunately, when surgery does not prove successful, alternative impotence treatments are still available, including the installation of an implant. Nevertheless, significant strides are being made in the surgical treatment of impotence, and surgical solutions to impotence can be expected to grow in importance in the future.

EXTERNAL VACUUM DEVICES

It has been said that nature abhors a vacuum. When a flaccid penis is surrounded by a vacuum, blood, in accordance with this age-old principle, is drawn into the erectile tissues and the penis will grow in size and rigidity, resulting in an erection. The erection can be maintained in this state for a period of time sufficient for intercourse by placing a specially designed tension band around the base of the penis that serves to keep blood trapped within the penis.

External vacuum devices are mechanical devices designed to provide an erection in this manner. For many years, such devices were largely purchased through sex or novelty shops or from mail order companies specializing in sexual items. One of the authors came across an external vacuum device for the first time some years ago in the window of a sleazy sex shop in the Soho district of London. In recent years, however, external vacuum devices have gained in medical respectability, and such devices are now recognized as a possibly effective impotence treatment option for some men. The better devices today are obtained only by medical prescription.

Osborn Medical Systems, Augusta, Georgia, a company that has pioneered the external vacuum device field since the 1960s, manufactures a product that incorporates a plastic vacuum chamber resembling a condom. The chamber is connected by a flexible plastic tube to a hand-held vacuum pump. Depending upon the model, the pump can be operated either by hand or by a small battery-driven motor. To use the device, the penis is inserted into the open end of the vacuum chamber and the vacuum applied. When the erection is obtained, the tension band is pushed from its position surrounding the base of the vacuum chamber to a position at the base of the penis.

External vacuum devices provide a simple, nominative, and relatively inexpensive means of obtaining an erection. The reported incidence of side effects among users is low. In cases of true psychological impotence, an external vacuum device can serve as a temporary expedient during the course of treatment. User success has been reported to be as high a 90 percent.

Disadvantages include complaints, by some patients, that the erections obtained are not of sufficient rigidity for satisfactory intercourse. Other complaints include impaired ejaculation and discomfort in use. Regarding the latter point, one patient used the phrase, "barbaric torture device." There is also a reported high patient dropout rate. External vacuum devices should not be used by some men with a history of leukemia, sickle-cell anemia, blood clotting problems, and penile injuries.

Simple rings that can be placed at various positions along the shaft of the penis in an attempt to sustain an erection are sometimes available from questionable sources. Such devices are usually ineffective. In the case of so-called "cock" rings, sometimes advertised in sex magazines, they can be dangerous. For example, after Roger appeared in the office with three permanent bends in his penis, it took an involved surgical procedure to literally straighten him out. Eventually, Roger had to have an implant to properly restore sexual function.

SUMMARY

At present, of the three approaches discussed in this chapter, the penile implant represents the most workable and permanent solution for an impotence problem for most patients. Patients have available several good choices as to type of implant. An overwhelming number of patients report satisfaction after having received an implant. Problems associated with implants are relatively infrequent.

Surgical approaches to the treatment of impotence, involving vascular surgery, are still at an early state of development. In time, such approaches can be expected to yield useful alternatives to penile implants in many more patients. There is also a role for external vacuum devices, especially in men who experience good results and wish to avoid more aggressive treatment.

TREATING IMPOTENCE WITH PSYCHOTHERAPY AND SEX THERAPY

This chapter describes the principal methods currently being used for the treatment of impotence presumably of a psychological origin. These treatments include traditional psychotherapy and more contemporary treatment methods commonly grouped under the term "sex therapy." Also discussed is how such treatments can provide needed support to men with impotence of known physical origin and their partners.

It should again be emphasized that no extensive treatment program for impotence that involves psychoanalysis or some form of sex therapy should be undertaken until the possibility of an identifiable physical cause is completely ruled out. Failure to do so could result in a delay in obtaining effective treatment, unnecessary emotional stress, and considerable expense. Any responsible psychotherapist or sex therapist will make this point clear to all prospective patients. However, if the condition is causing relationship problems, psychoanalysis can be very helpful.

In general, the number of accurate scientific studies of the effectiveness of psychological treatments for impotence has been limited. The studies that are available often reveal a mixed pattern of success. The chances for success are logically best in the case of men with impotence of a psychological origin and no evidence of any physical problem causing the impotence. It is also logical that some men with psychological impotence and only borderline physical problems may be helped to some extent.

USE OF TRADITIONAL PSYCHOTHERAPY

As observed in Chapter 2, traditional psychoanalytical theory originally attributed impotence to the existence of unconscious conflict arising from the incest taboo and various traumatic childhood sexual experiences. In time, the explanation was broadened to include other possible causes, such as repressed anger against a partner and general feelings of incompetence. The psychoanalytic process is intended to uncover these underlying experiences, and with this knowledge it is anticipated that the impotence problem will disappear.

The basic format employed in traditional one-on-one psychotherapy is familiar to most persons and need not be discussed here in depth. A man subject to impotence problems who elects such therapy can usually look forward to several preliminary 45- to 50-minute sessions with the therapist, devoted to taking a detailed personal history and to reviewing past and present physical and emotional problems. In subsequent sessions, the patient is encouraged to discuss freely, in an essentially unconstructed manner, memories of past events, relationships with others, personal fears, dreams, current conscious experiences, and so forth.

Therapy sessions continue on this basis indefinitely. In highly traditional therapy, sessions may occur at the rate of as many as four sessions per week. With other therapists the sessions may be scheduled at the rate of one per week. There is usually some time off during the course of the year to allow for the therapist's vacation periods.

Some therapists suggest that a period of at least two years is required before any tangible progress can be experienced, arguing that it takes at least that long for the patient to overcome inhibitions and freely confide to his therapist his most intimate personal feelings. According to traditional psychoanalytical theory, the patient gradually develops a strong dependence on the therapist during the course of the sessions. With the subsequent achievement of insight, the patient finds himself relieved of a wide spectrum of psychological problems, including impotence. In time, the patient is also able to function without the support of the therapist, and therefore eventually will be in a position to discontinue treatment. The entire process may take years.

The interpretation of dreams has been a key element in traditional psychotherapy. This is based on the belief that dreams provide access to important, but threatening, matters that are repressed by the conscious mind. Patients are encouraged to write down dream sequences promptly upon awakening for later discussion at therapy sessions. Various symbolic images appearing in dreams are believed to be representative of important psychological factors and are therefore of great significance in dream interpretation.

Current research on artificial intelligence systems, as employed in the computer field, suggests interesting insights in the functioning of the intelligence system of the human brain. This research raises some doubt as to the general area of dream interpretation. Artificial intelligence systems have a finite capacity, and thus are prone to disruption when computer electronic memory circuits are overloaded with information. The memory circuits of the human brain are also finite. Dreams could merely be a routine mechanism for the purging of extraneous information to make room for new information. Should this theory prove valid, it could follow that dreams hardly provide a window on the human mind. In fact, dreams might be somewhat analogous to the confused jumble of characters sometimes seen on computer displays, known to computer hackers as "garbage."

Can psychotherapy in practice actually help men with psychological impotence? The answer appears to be yes, although the process may prove torturous. In one report that appeared in medical literature in 1972, about one-fourth of a study group of men with impotence problems experienced some improvement after being in therapy at the rate of four sessions per week over a period of at least two years. Improvement was also experienced in about one-half of a group who had received less intensive therapy.

Given the high degree of personal commitment that is implied in undertaking any extensive program of psychotherapy, men with true psychological impotence are well advised to consider carefully their overall situation. Psychotherapy is designed to treat simultaneously a wide variety of problems. Under these circumstances, the use of psychotherapy for the treatment of impotence alone can prove unsuccessful on a cost-effective basis. On the other hand, a man with psychological impotence plus a wide variety of other emotional problems that are sufficiently serious to justify treatment might conclude that the overall benefits would make a program of psychotherapy worthwhile.

SENSATE FOCUS THERAPY

Variations exist in the treatment programs employing the sensate focus approach made popular by Masters and Johnson. Typically, such programs are short, but intensive, in nature and involve lengthy interactive discussions with sex therapists, education in sexual matters, and graduated sexual exercises. The educational component is intended to overcome misconceptions about sex, which are believed to contribute in some manner to inadequate sexual performance. The exercise component is designed to overcome the problem of performance anxiety. Most sensate focus therapy programs involve the active participation of male and female partners, usually a married couple, throughout the treatment process.

As discussed in Chapter 3, sensate focus therapy is largely a result of Masters and Johnson studies conducted during the 1960s. Most current sensate focus treatment programs today are heavily influenced by the original Masters and Johnson treatment model. The treatment was designed to deal with the sexual problems of both men and women and a variety of dysfunction problems. The original Masters and Johnson treatment model consisted of fourteen consecutive days of intensive therapy for both partners. Participants were encouraged to regard the experience as a vacation or retreat free from such day-to-day distractions as children and employment. Such conditions were believed to maximize the possibility of treatment success.

Couples participating in the program spent their first three days providing medical history, undergoing physical examinations, and participating in intensive discussions with an assigned male and female cotherapy team. By the third day, they were instructed to begin simple and nondemanding sexual exercises, but with all genital contact discouraged. On the fourth day, the participants received specific instructions for the remainder of the program tailored toward the particular problem to be overcome (impotence, premature ejaculation, and so forth). The remaining days of the program were largely devoted to sexual exercises conducted in private by the participating couple, but with the availability of the cotherapist team for active consultation and advice.

The key element in the general Masters and Johnson approach, as it is employed today, is the gradual and nondemanding nature of the prescribed sexual exercises. Initial exercises are typically limited to the simple stroking of nongenital body parts, such as the face and back. Genital contact, when finally established, proceeds from mild touching. The female partner is instructed to carefully avoid the verbal and nonverbal communication of personal sexual demands. When attempted intercourse seems propitious, the position with the female astride the male is prescribed, to minimize stress on the male. Use of other positions and attendance to the female's needs is suggested only during the advanced stages of the treatment program.

Brief mention should be made regarding the use of female surrogates, which has been sensationalized in the media. Use of such surrogates, at least by Masters and Johnson, has been largely limited to men subject to primary impotence. Such men, given their problem, often do not have an ongoing relationship with a female partner. Presumably, there is no effective way to help such men without provision for a surrogate. The use of surrogates obviously should be avoided unless the surrogate is very well trained and subject to the supervision of a qualified sex therapist.

Variations of the sensate focus approach involve departures from the original fourteen-day format, supplementing the treatment program with various elements derived from traditional psychotherapy, behavioral therapy, biofeedback, and hypnosis. Dr. Bernie Zilbergeld, a California-based sex therapist, has suggested a series of sexual exercises that emphasize the use of masturbation. Some of Zilbergeld's exercises, in this coauthor's opinion, appear to be bizarre. For example, in one suggested exercise, the patient is asked to compose a letter from the penis to its owner, expressing a series of grievances. Emphasis is placed in many of the suggested masturbation exercises on extended periods of self-stimulation and the delaying of ejaculation. This could result in prostate congestion and painful irritation.

How effective is sensate focus therapy? The original Masters and Johnson studies reported a success rate in the treatment of impotence in the range of approximately 60 to 70 percent. Stated another way, this implies failure in about one-third of the patients. The criteria for measuring success in the studies was fairly modest, being the ability to maintain an erection throughout intercourse at least 25 percent of the time. From a cost-benefit standpoint, successful sensate focus therapy appears to offer an advantage over traditional psychotherapy in the specific treatment of psychological impotence. Of course, it does not provide, as a by-product, the treatment of other problems of an emotional nature.

OTHER TREATMENTS

Various other treatments of a psychological nature have been attempted for impotence. One such approach is behavior therapy, which employs systematic conditioning techniques, with the intention of modifying some undesired aspect of human behavior. In the motion picture *A Clockwork Orange,* the general public was exposed to a provocative example of the use of behavior therapy in the treatment of antisocial behavior.

The treatment of impotence with behavior therapy generally revolves around some scheme to overcome performance anxiety. In the most common approach, known as desensitization, the patient is first encouraged to relax completely. Sometimes appropriate drugs are used to assist relaxation. The patient is then asked to imagine or actually view a series of sexual images. The images are arranged in order of increasing sexual explicitness, and are therefore intended to present increasing anxiety to the patient. No new image, however, is presented until the patient is able to cope with the previous image without anxiety.

The theory is that the patient, when ultimately desensitized to the most erotic and threatening sexual image in the series, will be able to perform with a partner in an actual sexual situation. One study has reported some degree of improvement in about three quarters of a group of men treated for impotence in this manner.

Biofeedback is a fairly recent concept that involves training individuals to control various bodily functions which are capable of being monitored in some appropriate manner, such as viewing images on a video screen. Biofeedback, for example, has been used with some degree of success in the treatment of hypertension. In this particular case, patients are trained in appropriate techniques to control their blood pressure levels, with continuous measurements of blood pressure providing an immediate indication of the degree of success in achieving control.

The use of biofeedback in the treatment of impotence has typically involved the imagining or actual viewing of erotic, sexual images, accompanied by the continuous monitoring of penile physical dimensions to indicate erectile success. If the treatment proves successful, the patient, over a period of time, is expected to gradually gain some degree of control over the ability to achieve an erection and is able to carry over this control into an actual sexual situation. Studies to date of the use of biofeedback training in the treatment of impotence are inconclusive, but generally discouraging.

It should be noted that skepticism does exist about the effectiveness of techniques that involve observation of erectile response to the viewing of erotic images. During the cold war, a testing procedure was developed by governmental authorities in the former Czechoslovakia intended to unmask men claiming to be gay in order to avoid compulsory military duty. Men were presumed to be draft evaders when there was no indication of erection upon viewing images of a homosexual nature. Attempts have been made to employ the Czechoslovakian device in the United States in situations involving individuals suspected of child abuse. It should be obvious that any such test would be meaningless in the case of a man with physical erectile dysfunction. There is also reason to suspect that many men without physical response would fail to have erections under such uncomfortable and unnatural conditions.

Hypnotherapy has sometimes been attempted in the treatment of impotence. Hypnotism is an old technique that has been used on occasion for legitimate medical purposes. On the other hand, hypnotism has all too often been the province of the quack or stage performer. Hypnotherapy revolves around the concept of posthypnotic suggestion. While in a hypnotic state, some desired medical response is communicated to the patient. If the treatment is successful, the patient will later respond in the desired manner.

Hypnotherapy has sometimes been used in the treatment of psychological impotence, in combination with traditional psychotherapy. The inducement of a hypnotic state has been used to identify deeply repressed experiences that may underlie the impotence problem. Attempts have also been made to induce erections in patients under hypnosis. Individual cases have been reported of successful treatment of impotence using hypnotherapy. However, conclusive scientific evidence demonstrating the positive value of hypnotherapy is lacking to date.

In general, behavior therapy, biofeedback training, and hypnotherapy should be approached with caution. Behavior therapy and biofeedback training should be regarded as essentially experimental techniques at this time. While hypnotherapy has existed for some time, the lack of serious ongoing scientific research in this field is grounds for concern. Men with impotence problems are advised to steer clear of such treatments, unless offered under the auspices of a highly regarded medical center and by practitioners with verifiable credentials.

Counseling for Support Purposes

Emotional factors are important in all forms of erectile dysfunction, including both impotence of a physical nature, as well as psychological. In many instances, a urologist treating a patient with physical impotence is able merely by simple office visit counseling to provide sufficient support on how to deal with the associated emotional problems. In some cases, the urologist may recommend concurrent treatment by appropriate psychological specialists. This is often the case with patients with coexistent problems such as alcoholism, drug abuse, and dysfunctional personal relationships. The urologist may also recommend that the partner receive counseling.

One area where counseling can be of great value is educating partners as to what is normal sexual behavior and response. Unfortunately, there is widespread ignorance as to what is sexually normal, and this can result in unrealistic expectations and performance anxiety. Some key areas that can be addressed during such counseling include the normal frequency of intercourse between partners in stabile relationships, how long does it typically take either partner to achieve an orgasm during intercourse, how long is it reasonable to expect a man to be able to sustain an erection, how long should it take a man to again obtain an erection following ejaculation, the relationship between sexual performance and age, whether masturbation and oral sex are a normal form of sexual activity, and what is normal when it comes to sexual fantasies. Clearing up misconceptions regarding these and other questions often serves to improve personal relationships and sometimes actual sexual performance. It may also help enhance the intimacy and pleasure of sex for both partners, even in cases where a problem of physical impotence exists.

TREATING OTHER MALE SEXUAL DYSFUNCTION PROBLEMS

Although this book deals primarily with the impotence problem, other forms of male sexual dysfunction can be as troubling to both the afflicted man and his partner. In many cases, such problems may lead to erectile dysfunction of either a physical or psychological nature.

TREATING PREMATURE EJACULATION

After impotence, premature ejaculation is the male sexual problem that receives the most attention. Some estimates

191

indicate that as many as 30 million men have at some time experienced at least a single premature ejaculation episode. When such episodes become increasingly common and reach a point where they take place about 25 percent of the time, it makes sense to consult a urologist. This advice is especially relevant in the case of an older man who has previously never found premature ejaculation to be a problem.

As discussed in Chapter 5, premature ejaculation may be caused by a prostate infection (prostatitis). How to recognize whether you have such an infection was also discussed. Prostate infections, however, can be quite difficult to detect, and any symptoms that you may observe may be actually only that of a low-grade urinary tract infection. It is also a fact that a man can harbor a low-grade infection without knowing it. Such men may feel generally rundown but may exhibit little in the way of overt symptoms. Actually, premature ejaculation may be the only symptom. As a consequence, it is a good idea, especially for older men, to have frequent prostate examinations to detect a possible prostate infection or a more serious problem.

A full examination requires the physician to probe the gland through the anus, and also to exert pressure, with massage, to force a small quantity of fluid through the penis. The fluid is then examined in the laboratory to make a definitive determination of infection. The laboratory procedure includes looking for the presence of any bacteria and puslike areas under the microscope and the culturing of the fluid in a nutrient-rich medium to determine the type of microorganism causing problems. As the process is unpleasant to many men, ultrasonic devices are being developed to permit noninvasive scanning of the prostate. Ultrasonic scanning, while potentially useful, will not substitute for the fluid-collecting process.

One reason why the prostate is subject to persistent infection is that its internal structure allows any disease-causing microorganisms that manage to reach the gland to collect and build up in numbers. Due to the lack of good drainage, the body's natural immune system cannot easily overcome the invasion. Frequent massage of the prostate gland encourages drainage, but it is obviously impractical.

There are things, however, that you can do to prevent prostate infections from taking place in the first place. The coliform bacteria that cause most prostate infections most often reach the gland by traveling through the urethra. Such bacteria are normally present in large numbers in the colon and therefore are present in fecal matter. It follows that you can minimize the chances of infection by carefully washing your hands following a bowel movement. Coliform bacteria can also be transmitted during sexual relations. This is another reason for practicing safe sex.

Most prostate infections are easily cured by antibiotics. Bactrim and Septra are the trade names of the sulfa medications most commonly used. During treatment, the prescribed drug must be taken for the full amount of time specified, and alcohol should be avoided, as it often interferes with the action of many antibiotics. If it does not cause discomfort, sex is actually helpful while being treated for a prostate infection. You should, however, wear a condom to avoid passing the infection back and forth with your partner. Treatment requires a follow-up prostate examination to make sure the infection has been fully eliminated.

After treatment, premature ejaculation should disappear, assuming the infection was the real cause of the problem. As a by-product, after treatment many men feel much healthier, as they have eliminated something that had been adversely affecting their overall system. Curing a prostate infection, however, may have no effect on an impotence problem.

If a physical problem does not exist, sex therapy or more psychotherapy can be tried. In treating premature ejaculation with sex therapy, a variety of approaches are used, depending upon the therapist, including masturbation exercises. The Masters and Johnson approach for the treatment of premature ejaculation, in its early stages, is identical to the one used for treating impotence (see Chapter 9). At some point in the treatment, the female partner is directed to assume a "training" position. In this position, the woman is seated with her legs apart and her back pressed against the headboard of the bed. Her partner lies on his back with his pelvic area facing upward between her legs. In this position, she has easy access to her partner's penis and can conveniently employ a penile "squeeze" technique designed to retard ejaculation.

Unfortunately, the squeeze and other techniques often do not work. Too-frequent use of such techniques may also result in prostate irritation. In such cases, penile injection therapy may be helpful. With the injection and subsequent extended erection, the patient with a psychological premature ejaculation problem is able to achieve vaginal penetration regardless of when ejaculation actually occurs. As success of this nature raises the patient's confidence and helps to overcome performance anxiety, the problem may eventually disappear.

In the last few years, fluoxetine, a drug sold under the trade name Prozac and used mainly for treating depression, has been shown to be highly effective in treating premature ejaculation. At the Morganstern Clinic, Atlanta, Georgia, over 90 percent of the men that we have treated with Prozac for premature ejaculation have been greatly helped. Prozac is known to work on serotonin, a substance found in the brain that acts as a neurotransmitter. A link exits between serotonin nerve pathways and the nerve receptors for the female sex hormones that control menstruation in women. It is, therefore, revealing that Prozac has been shown in some recent studies to help women with premenstrual syndrome. It could be that Prozac works in a similar manner in connection with the physical mechanism that controls ejaculation in men.

Warning! A variety of quack remedies for premature ejaculation, such as "numbing creams," are available. These remedies are by and large useless—some potentially dangerous—and they should be avoided.

TREATING RETROGRADE EJACULATION

When retrograde ejaculation is due to sphincter muscle damage following prostate surgery or accidental injury, the condition might presumably be treated with suitable reconstructive surgical procedures intended to strengthen the defect in the valving mechanism that is allowing seminal fluid to pass into the bladder, rather than through the penis. There has been little incentive to develop surgical techniques of this nature, as retrograde ejaculation does not represent a threat to health, and an alternative exists for dealing with the problem faced by men who wish to have children. In the small number of cases where retrograde ejaculation can be traced to the taking of the drug thioridazine, it, of course, may be possible to shift to an effective alternate drug for needed emotional control.

Fortunately, most men who suffer from retrograde ejaculation following prostate surgery are of the age when children are no longer desired. When the problem results from a physical injury, it is more likely that the victim is a younger man desiring children. In such cases, the ability to father children can be achieved by collecting the first passage of urine from the bladder following ejaculation. The sperm can then be filtered out of the urine in the laboratory and used to artificially inseminate the female partner. Although the esthetics can be troubling to some persons, the approach is effective as long as there is no defect with the sperm. As to any doubt that sperm can survive the brief period of immersion in urine, consider the ability of sperm to overcome chemical and physical barriers presented in many forms of birth control.

There is a possibility that the lack of visible ejaculate may trouble some men, or even their partners. This could be the case with a man who feels compelled to feign orgasm, out of a mistaken belief that its absence somehow indicates personal failure. This is a problem to be solved by greater communication between the partners, and possibly by counseling.

TREATING EJACULATORY FAILURE

Treatment of the anorgasmic male has not received the attention that it deserves, due to the fairly rare occurrence of persistent ejaculatory failure. This is unfortunate, as effective treatment can be difficult to accomplish while, at the same time, the condition is very troubling to afflicted men and their partners.

In treating failure to ejaculate, it is logical to first check to see whether the patient is currently taking any of the drugs listed in Appendix A as being linked to the problem and, if possible, substitute an alternative drug. The next step would be to investigate the possibility of a hormonal or neurological abnormality and to treat any such condition uncovered whenever possible. There is little difficulty in identifying the cause of the problem when there has been a recent major spinal injury. When there is nerve damage from an old forgotten injury of childhood, identification is more difficult.

As a result of continuing research in rehabilitation medicine, it is no longer hopeless when a man with a spinal injury and his partner want children. A technique now exists in which electrodes are implanted to critical nerve areas controlling ejaculation. When a small electrical charge is applied, ejaculation results.

The ejaculate is then collected and used to artificially inseminate the female partner. Electroejaculation will not result in the pleasurable sensations of orgasm, but the ability to have children will greatly enrich the lives of couples faced with these unfortunate circumstances. It is most likely that research in the general area will ultimately lead to workable treatment methods for all anorgasmic men.

When a physical cause cannot be identified, and the problem is presumed to be psychological in nature, sex therapy may prove useful. Masters and Johnson report a high degree of success in the treatment of the problem. The Masters and Johnson treatment for ejaculatory failure, as in the case for premature ejaculation, follows the same general format, in the beginning, as in the treatment of impotence. At an intermediate point in the program, the male partner is encouraged to masturbate to ejaculation in the presence of his partner. Subsequently, the female partner is expected to manipulate the penis to a point approaching ejaculatory inevitability, then rapidly mount the male and position the penis in her vagina just prior to ejaculation. The initial manipulation of the penis and the pelvic thrusting after vaginal penetration by the female should be performed in a "demanding" manner. With patience and repeated practice, this approach is expected to result in an eventual resolution of the problem.

TREATING PRIAPISM

Priapism is always an emergency medical procedure. As a result, men at higher risk, such as victims of sickle-cell anemia, are well advised to be aware of the possibility. It is also important for such men to insist upon treatment by a urologist when seeking treatment in a hospital emergency room. Men taking any of the drugs listed in Appendix A as being linked to priapism should also follow this advice.

The treatment of priapism is essentially the same as that described in Chapter 7 in connection with the treatment of a prolonged erection that may occur in penile injection therapy. It includes the injection of adrenalin (epinephrine), and possibly drawing blood from the penis. The prospects for successful treatment are obviously much greater for men with a prolonged erection after a penile injection, as such men are under the continuing care of a urologist, know what to expect, and have rapid access to a specialist in an emergency.

TREATING PEYRONIE'S DISEASE

Scarring of the penis characteristic of Peyronie's disease will often disappear on its own, in time, leaving no lasting problems. This can occur as much as 50 percent of the time. For this reason, when the visible symptoms are first noted and do not cause a problem, a urologist may suggest carefully observing the situation for a reasonable period of time.

Before recommending surgery, many urologists will first suggest trying some form of noninvasive treatment. These can include the use of vitamin E therapy, steroid injections, and ultrasound. Unfortunately, these treatments are not always effective. Vitamin E therapy, which has, in some instances, reduced scar tissue in various parts of the body, is tried for a period of about twelve months. Treatment with potassium p-aminobenzoate, a drug sold under the trade name Potaba, is often conducted concurrently. This drug, which is available in tablets, has been most often used in the treatment of various dermatological diseases. Experimental work is underway on treatments that involve the injection of certain enzymes known to dissolve scar tissues.

If more aggressive treatment is necessary, the choice is some form of surgery. Most surgical procedures involve at least the tightening of penile skin over the affected area. The Nesbit procedure, which uses this approach, is most often used and is suitable for patients with moderate penile deformation who fortunately still enjoy normal erectile capability. More complicated procedures, involving the cutting away of scar tissue and skin grafts, are employed when there is greater penile curvature. A penile implant may be required when there is a simultaneous impotence problem. This can be the case when a significant growth of plaque into the interior of the penis makes erection impossible.

TREATING PAINFUL EJACULATION

Usually, painful ejaculation is easily treated with antibiotics when the problem is due to a prostate infection. (Treatment of prostate infections is described in connection with premature ejaculation.)

If no physical cause can be found, it may be assumed that the problem is psychological. If the problem persists over an extended period, psychotherapy may be indicated.

Painful ejaculation and blood in the urine, also a symptom of prostate infection, should always be medically investigated. The reason is not only the possible long-range consequences of prostate infection, but also the very real possibility that these problems could result in loss of desire, performance anxiety, and even psychological impotence.

TREATING LACK OF DESIRE

Lack of desire obviously is a psychological problem, but one that can very well have a physical cause. It is therefore advisable to first determine whether a physical problem exists. A problem may be the taking of one of the drugs listed in Appendix A. When there are hormonal abnormalities, such as elevated prolactin or depressed testosterone levels, the problem may disappear with appropriate hormonal therapy. When lack of desire is the psychological response to impotence caused by physical factors, the logical approach is the appropriate treatment of the impotence problem. If lack of desire is associated with depression, it is advisable to promptly investigate the depression in its own right.

Simple family counseling may be helpful when there is reason to believe the problem is purely psychological and results from some failure in a stable and mutually desired relationship between two partners. If the problem is more deep seated, appropriate psychotherapy may be required, especially when there is depression for which there is no apparent physical explanation.

TREATING PERFORMANCE ANXIETY

Performance anxiety is another example of a psychological problem that can often have a physical cause. Treating the physical problem often overcomes the performance anxiety.

For example, Norman, age 55, became increasingly anxious after repeated episodes of premature ejaculation. He feared the possible ridicule of his much younger wife. Eventually he avoided all sexual activity. Norman's problem was due to a prostate infection. When this was cured, his fears as to proper performance were overcome, and normal sexual activities were resumed.

When it is concluded, after a full examination, that performance anxiety in a given case has no physical basis, it does not follow that the psychological factors, apparently at work, are deep seated or result from traumatic experiences in early childhood. It is very possible that the problem may result from lack of proper sex education. Some modest counseling may prove to be the solution to the anxiety problem.

For example, gross misconceptions may be taking a toll. Sam, a 25-year-old patient, was highly fearful of entering into any relationship with a woman. There was nothing wrong with Sam physically. During the course of the examination, Sam asked whether anything could be done to increase the size of his penis. His nonerect penis actually measured 5 inches, well above average. Sam had been avoiding women largely because he feared being ridiculed for a nonexistent physical abnormality.

Mistaken expectations about sex can also underlie performance anxiety. If there is any truth to the suggestion that the greater assertiveness of women associated with the feminist movement is contributing to male sexual dysfunction, it will be most likely felt in this connection. One very undesirable aspect of pornography is that it tends to reinforce the many incorrect ideas about sexual performance first learned in teenage conversations. Exactly what is involved in "satisfying" a woman may be very misunderstood. Although the simultaneous orgasm of both partners is actually not all that frequent, failure for this to occur can result in anxiety in some men. Other men may become very anxious over their failure to perform as well as male actors they have seen in X-rated films. Actually, such films are typically produced over an extended period of time, due to the limited capabilities of the actors. What is seen is really an illusion.

Penile injection therapy has a role in treating performance anxiety in patients with no identifiable physical problem. Martin, an unmarried psychologist in good health, suffered great anxiety at the beginning of new sexual relationships. Despite counseling, he had not been able to overcome an excessive fear of failure. His solution was an injection prior to the first attempt at sex in a new relationship. The resulting successful performance in each instance gave him the confidence to continue the relationship without resorting to further injections.

Sex therapy plays an important role when the psychological factors involved in performance anxiety are deep seated. More intensive psychotherapy may very well be indicated when the patient's emotional problems are found to include not only anxiety over sexual performance, but also an abnormal level of anxiety about other aspects of behavior.

Treating Inadequate Penile Size

As discussed in Chapter 3, some men are unable to adjust to having what they consider to be inadequately sized penises, despite psychological counseling. For a man with this problem, operative procedures have been developed that result in an increase in the visible length of the penis or enhance its girth. Both operations, if desired, can be performed at the same time.

The operation used to increase penis length is based on the fact that the unseen portion of the penis is at least as long as the portion that is normally visible. A web of tissue exists between the underside of the penis and the scrotum which serves to arch the hanging penis outward. When this arch is released, the visible penis will increase as much as 50.8 centimeters (2.0 inches in length), with the average increase in the 25.4- to 38.1-centimeter (1.0- to 1.5-inch) range. The operation for enhancing penile girth employs the process known as liposuction in which fat is sucked out of some other area of the body and deposited under the skin around the penis. This process results in a gain of about 2.54 centimeters (about 1 inch) in the circumference of the penis.

Both operations require a one-night hospital stay. There is a slight amount of discomfort on the first day following surgery, with the pain typically easily controlled with oral medications. The surgical sutures are removed eight days following surgery. There is some swelling that typically lasts about two weeks. Sexual relations can be resumed after a period of up to six weeks. No patient treated at the Morganstern Clinic has reported erectile dysfunction due to these treatments.

Treating Other Problems

An intractable foreskin is easily treated by circumcision. Prostate irritation is treated by educating the patient as to a proper pattern of sexual activities. This includes avoiding extended stimulus of the penis not followed by ejaculation, not using coitus interruptus (pulling out) for birth control, and not engaging in short periods of excessive sexual activity. Extended periods of sexual abstinence should also be avoided. When this is not possible, masturbation is advised. In the case of men who object to masturbation, periodic prostate massage by a urologist to relieve excess build of prostate fluid is an option.

CHAPTER 11

GETTING HELP AND WHAT IT WILL COST

A patient being treated for an impotence problem once was said to have remarked: "Doctor, it's not the performance anxiety that's really bothering me. It's the payment anxiety."

This story, while probably apocryphal, is nevertheless revealing of a very legitimate problem. Treatment of male sexual dysfunction does cost money. The costs, moreover, can clearly be a serious consideration to the typical patient, particularly when a penile implant is the best solution. Very often, a man requiring an implant is at an age when limited family financial resources must be allocated among a variety of pressing demands. These demands may include the cost of tuition for university-age children, the support of aging parents, the expenses for treating other medical problems, or savings for retirement. The need for treatment may occur at the very time when the patient had hoped to have something left over for such reasonable pleasures of life as international travel, a vacation home, or even frequent meals out. Under the circumstances, it is not uncommon for the patient to feel guilty about spending money on something as "selfish" as personal sexual pleasure.

It is important, therefore, to be aware that the actual out-of-pocket costs may prove to be less than feared. Total treatment costs may also be subject to some degree of control, through careful planning by the patient. Furthermore, the costs should be weighed against the benefits that are not limited to just the patient's sexual pleasure. After weighing all the factors, this could be one of the best investments that the patient could make for his entire family.

The purpose of this chapter is to provide reasonable estimates of the total overall cost of obtaining help. In most circumstances, this involves the net total cost to the patient after any reimbursements from medical insurance programs. Many patients may also be in the position to reduce the total cost by taking advantage of the deductions allowable under current federal and state income tax codes.

Costs shown in this chapter are typical of those prevailing in mid-1993 in one large American urban area. Costs, of course, vary throughout the country. Unfortunately, medical costs, in general, have been continually rising for the past several decades, and there is no reason to anticipate this trend will stop. You are cautioned, therefore, to update the information given, and make reasonable allowances for the pattern of costs prevailing in your local community.

Special note: As this is written, the current Washington administration is in the process of developing a comprehensive national health plan. The plan is expected to be unveiled in late 1993. In the normal course of events, any plan, as initially submitted, will probably be subject to modification before being enacted into law. There is, therefore, no way of knowing exactly how any major change in the American health care system will impact on future costs and insurance coverage for the treatment of male sexual dysfunction. As male sexual dysfunction is now widely recognized as a legitimate public health problem, it is reasonable to believe that adequate insurance coverage will be available under any new program. Should you initiate treatment following the effective date of the new national health plan, you should discuss its financial implications with your health care provider.

ESTIMATING THE TOTAL COST

Costs for the treatment of male sexual dysfunction logically fall into two general categories. First, there are the charges that will be incurred in diagnosing the problem. Second, there are the expenses that will be incurred in treatment.

Costs of Diagnosing the Problem

As is the practice of all physicians, urologists specializing in male sexual dysfunction charge for their professional time and any special tests or other procedures that may be required. The number of visits and tests that may be required, of course, depend upon the patient and the problem. As noted in Chapter 6, a reliable diagnosis of an impotence problem can often be achieved in two or three visits. The following is an example of the charges that were incurred by one patient in arriving at a diagnosis of his problem.

Item	Charges
Initial office visit and detailed examination	$92
Follow-up visits—$40 per visit	80
Blood tests—testosterone and prolactin levels	250
Penile blood flow test	150
Penile snap gage test—two at $45 per test	90
Urinalysis—two at $12 each	24
Total billed to patient	$686

The charge shown in the example for blood testing may seem excessive compared to the relatively modest charge incurred for routine blood testing in an annual physical examination. The high cost reflects the complex analytical procedures that are performed in the laboratory when determining the hormonal levels. In some instances, the cost for blood testing during an initial visit proves to be somewhat less when a broad spectrum of blood characteristics is not indicated.

In the example shown, the patient's impotence problem was found to be largely due to an abnormally low level of testosterone. The total cost incurred by the patient in reaching an accurate diagnosis is fairly typical for this type of condition.

Total cost of diagnosis, of course, varies depending upon the circumstances. If a corpora cavernosagram, for example, is indicated, a typical charge is $265. Costs can mount when nocturnal penile tumescence (NPT) monitoring is necessitated. Some insurance companies insist upon this procedure, often without any real justification. When this is the case, a charge in the $600–650 range is not unusual, and the procedure can extend over three nights. When home testing using a portable monitor is acceptable, the cost typically is at about the $200- per-night level. When the simple snap gauge test is sufficient, the cost, as indicated in the preceding example, is typically about $90.

Costs of Treating the Problem

Typical charges that are often incurred in the treatment of impotence are shown in the accompanying table. From this information it should be possible to arrive at a reasonable preliminary estimate of what treatment might cost you, depending on the nature of the problem and taking into consideration geographical variations in your part of the country.

Treatment, of course, might turn out to cost virtually nothing, should the problem be easily solved by switching to alternative drugs for the control of a high blood pressure problem. The cost for treatment is generally moderate when hormone or drug therapy is indicated. Obviously, penile implants and other treatments that necessitate surgical procedures are considerably more expensive. Where a penile implant is indicated, total costs can vary over a fairly wide range, depending on the type of implant selected by the patient and options as to hospitalization.

Representative Treatment Charges[1]

Item	Charge
1:Hormone and Drug Therapy	
Regular office visits—per visit	$ 40

---

1 Mid-1993.

Office testosterone injection	15–20
Testosterone pellet implant	500–550
Office papaverine injection	88–85
Office prostaglandin E_1 injection	300
Home papaverine injection	15–20
Home prostaglandin E_1 injection	50–70
Yohimbine—daily home dosage	1.25–$1.50

1:Treatments Necessitating Surgical Procedures
Penile implant

Cost of prosthesis	$6,000
Urologist's surgery fee[2]	4,000
Anesthesia—fee and supplies	2,000
Hospital—use of surgery and recovery facilities, room charge, and drugs	6,000

Other surgical procedures[3]

Phalloplasty for correction of penile angulation	725
Peyronie's disease plaque removal	930
Penile prosthesis repair	$3,000–3,500

Hormone and Drug Therapy[2]

As noted in Chapter 7, patients have several treatment options with testosterone therapy.[3] If the patient chooses to have testosterone injected by the physician during monthly office visits, annual treatment cost would normally be in the $450–500 range, including physician's fees and drug cost.

---

2 Inflatable implant (usually includes office follow-up).
3 Urologist's professional fee.

The cost will be cut to about half when the patient is willing to inject himself at home. Should the implantation of testosterone pellets under the skin be preferred, the typical cost for the entire procedure, with a sufficient number of pellets to be effective in most patients for about one year, would be about $525.

Determining the annual cost of penile injection therapy for impotence is more complicated. There is an initial cost, incurred for the series of office visits during which correct dosage level is determined experimentally, and the patient is carefully trained in proper procedures. The initial cost would include the charge for injections and the normal office visit charge. Subsequently, the patient can inject himself at home, using syringes obtained at the urologist's office which are prefilled with the proper amount of the drug. Alternatively, the patient may fill syringes at home, using a bottle of the drug supplied by the urologist. It is necessary to refrigerate the drug, whether supplied in prefilled syringes or in a bottle.

The cost of penile injection therapy is affected by the type of drug prescribed. When using prefilled syringes of papaverine, a cost in the $15–20 range might be incurred each time sexual activities were desired. If the drug of preference is prostaglandin E_1, the cost per home injection with prefilled injections might be in the $50–70 range. When the patient chooses to fill syringes at home, he will normally incur a cost of about $250 per bottle for papaverine and about three times as much for prostaglandin E1. Exactly how long the bottle will last obviously depends on the patient's dosage requirements, which can range from 0.1 to 0.4 cubic centimeters per patient, and on the frequency of sexual activities. In general, patients using papaverine incur an annual cost of about $500. Those using prostaglandin E_1 incur an annual cost of about $1,750. The greater cost of prostaglandin E_1, however, can be justified by its higher degree of effectiveness and greater control over the length of time an erection is desired.

When use of yohimbine is indicated, a cost will be incurred typically in the $1.25–1.50 range for the necessary daily dosage of the drug. As such, the annual cost for treatment might be at about the $500 level. When trazodone is prescribed, along with yohimbine, the annual cost will be somewhat higher.

Surgical Treatments

The first thing to consider in estimating the cost of a penile implant is the selection of a prosthesis. The advantages and disadvantages of the more common devices on the market are discussed in Chapter 8. The more complicated inflatable implants naturally cost the most to purchase and install. A top-of-the-line inflatable prosthesis typically is available for about $6,000. The fee to insert the device typically would be around $4,000. In contrast, the costs for obtaining a semirigid prosthesis and for insertion would typically be about one-half of that amount.

A second major factor that determines the total cost of a penile implant is the choice as to where the insertion procedure will take place. Depending upon the patient, there may be a choice between insertion on an inpatient basis at a hospital, insertion on an outpatient basis at a hospital, and insertion on an outpatient basis in a clinical facility. In general, anybody using a hospital's facilities is considered an inpatient and is charged full price for room and board if an overnight stay is involved. Given average prevailing rates for a semiprivate room, an implant inpatient might incur a charge of about $1,200 for a three-day hospital stay. Total room charges, however, could be cut to about $150 when the implant procedure is done in a hospital on an outpatient basis. Clinical patients are treated in a physician's office that is equipped with surgical facilities or at an ambulatory "surgicenter." Implant patients normally avoid all room charges when treated in a clinical facility.

In addition to room charges, there are also potential cost savings to outpatients treated at clinics. Such patients normally avoid hospital charges for surgical and recovery facilities and anesthesia fees and supplies. They are also usually charged at lower rates for drugs.

Given the various options, the overall current cost for a penile implant could range from as low as $10,000 to as high as $20,000. The lower end of the range might apply in the case of a patient requesting a semirigid implant that could be inserted in a clinic and on an outpatient basis. The higher end would apply to a patient requesting an inflatable implant and electing insertion as a hospital inpatient.

Saving money is not the only factor that a patient should consider when reviewing his options as to where insertion of an implant should take place. In making a decision, important factors to consider include the patient's general medical condition, his ability to withstand pain and discomfort, and convenience. Inpatient treatment does offer definite advantages with regard to the control of complications, the minimization of pain, and ensuring patient compliance with postoperative instructions. On the other hand, there are many individuals who greatly dislike spending any time in a hospital and very much prefer to recuperate in the privacy of their homes. The chance of postoperative infection is also greater in a hospital, due to the frequent presence of infectious bacteria in the hospital environment.

It is difficult to generalize as to the costs of other surgical procedures. At the low end of the spectrum are the relatively modest fees for the repairing of problems associated with Peyronie's disease. Surgery to remove an arterial blockage or to correct a leak in the veins carrying blood away from the penis, however, constitutes major medical procedures that typically result in significant charges for surgery and hospitalization. The total cost for either type of surgical procedures might be as high as $20,000.

External Vacuum Erection Devices

The cost of a vacuum erection device that is obtained under medical prescription varies depending upon the manufacturer and the individual design features. The cost can be in the $400–500 range, with the lower end for a device in which the vacuum is achieved by use of a hand pump and the higher end for a device that employs a battery-operated pump. The devices occasionally require servicing, but manufacturers typically provide warranties that cover any failure of the key components.

Sex Therapy

Sex therapy is usually billed on an hourly basis, with the charge varying significantly depending upon the academic training, general reputation, and geographical location of the therapist. Medical psychiatrists certified by the American Board of Psychiatry and Neurology typically command higher fees than do clinical psychologists with Ph.D.s. Other therapists with lesser credentials usually charge less. Fees charged in major urban areas are usually much higher than those in smaller cities. At present, fees charged by psychiatrists throughout the United States average about $125 per "hour." The "hour" is typically 50 minutes. Psychologist fees average about $100 per hour. Fees for other therapists can be as low as $25 per hour.

Intensive traditional psychotherapy can require as many as three sessions per week and possibly extend over a period of years. At the $125 rate charged by psychiatrists, this could result in an annual charge of about $20,000. At one session per week, the charge could add up to about $6,500 per year. Under some circumstances, it may be possible to reduce costs by obtaining treatment through a local mental health center, where there is some adjustment based on ability to pay.

Intensive therapy of the Masters and Johnson type, that takes place over a short time, is usually billed on an overall treatment program basis. The total cost is typically quite expensive, especially when treatment takes place on a residence basis and results in travel and lodging expense in addition to the actual treatment expense.

WHAT WILL INSURANCE PAY?

Insurance Company Attitudes

It is no secret that the ability to obtain medical services is increasingly dependent on the existence of a cooperative third party that is willing to pick up a major share of the tab. Such third parties include private insurance carriers, union health and welfare organizations, and publicly supported programs such as the Medicare system. Fortunately, most third parties to date have exhibited a reasonably enlightened view toward coverage of male sexual dysfunction.

Medical insurance is a difficult subject, given the large number of individual insurance carriers, the many different plans that are offered, and the "fine print" characteristics of most insurance policies. This is also an area where considerable change can be anticipated whenever a national health program makes its appearance. At present, claims submitted in connection with a physician's diagnosis of impotence or other types of dysfunction are approved by the typical claim examiner, unless there is a specific exclusion of this type of claim in the applicable policy. Many policies, however, exclude claims for "routine" visits to physicians' offices or visits that are "not medically necessary." Refusal to reimburse a claim for the diagnosis of an impotence problem, on the grounds that the physician's services are not medically necessary, is unlikely in view of the close linkage between dysfunction and diabetes, arteriosclerosis, and other serious diseases.

Claims for the treatment of impotence that involve hormonal and drug therapy are also usually reimbursed without too much difficulty. Men requiring testosterone supplementation may be subject to a variety of recognized medical problems, in addition to impotence, such as serious loss of physical vigor and muscular atrophy. Insurance companies have also raised little objection to penile injection therapy.

Individuals who have specific coverage in their insurance policies for the treatment of mental and nervous disorders usually do not experience too much difficulty in obtaining reimbursement for at least part of the cost of psychological and sex therapy. Many insurance policies, however, still do not provide adequate coverage in this area, with a $1,000 annual limitation very common. In some cases, the cost per visit and the number of visits to therapists are subject to significant limitations. Carriers are also known to pressure policy holders to utilize the services of therapists who bill at lower hourly rates.

Reimbursement of the cost of a penile implant is a matter of obvious concern. The accompanying table summarizes the current situation. The information shown is, by necessity, general in nature. Plans vary from company to company and are constantly changing.

REPRESENTATIVE INSURANCE COVERAGE OF PENILE IMPLANT CLAIMS

Plan or Carrier Category	Typical Coverage
Blue Cross/Blue Shield	Coverage is generally good. Plans offered under the Blue Cross/Blue Shield name, however, do vary throughout the United States and will occasionally change. In some instances, regional groups may exclude male sexual dysfunction. As a result, it is best to verify coverage before initiating any major treatment program.
Commercial Group Plans (plans available to type that are provided through employees or members well-known national insurance of affinity groups)	Coverage in most plans of this type that are provided through carriers such as Prudential, for example, is generally good. Plans occasionally change, often with minimum prior notice.
Commercial Individual Plans	Coverage is generally good. Many plans, however, are subject to high deductibles. Restrictive waiting periods for eligibility are also quite common.
Self-funded Employer Plans	Fair to good coverage, depending upon the company. Exclusion of dysfunction is rare. The professional staffs of in-house company clinics are often important influences in approving coverage.
Health Maintenance Organizations (HMOs)	Coverage is generally only poor to fair. Many HMOs limit or exclude specific types of prostheses and/or limit reimbursement to a fixed percentage of total cost.

Union Health and Welfare Plans	Large unions that operate on a national basis usually offer good coverage. Coverage can be only poor to fair with smaller unions and independent bargaining units. Elective surgery is very often not covered in the contracts of most small unions.
Plans for Federal, State, and Local Government Employees and the U.S. Postal Service	Coverage varies between individual employee groups, but is generally not generous. Dysfunction is often specifically excluded. A few plans do offer good coverage.
CHAMPUS (Civilian Health and Medical Programs of the United Services)	Coverage in most existing plans covering retired armed forces personnel and dependents of armed forces personnel has become more generous. Penile implants are now covered in cases where physical impotence can be demonstrated.
Veterans Administration	Coverage is possible and typically generous when a case can be made that the treatment is necessary for the rehabilitation of a service connected disability.
Workers' Compensation	State-operated workers' compensation programs usually provide excellent coverage for dysfunction problems that can be demonstrated to have a job-related origin. In most instances, this would mean a physical injury sustained on the job.
Medicare	Coverage of male sexual dysfunction is excellent, both with respect to diagnosis and treatment. As a national coverage policy for impotence exists, locally designated Medicare carriers are bound to the current favorable national policy. All claims, of course, are subject to standard Medicare deductibles, which can be expected to rise in the future.

Medicaid	Existing federal law does permit coverage under individual state programs. Coverage, however, varies considerably between states and should be verified in all instances.
Automobile and Public Liability Plans	Coverage depends upon the ability of the accident victim to demonstrate wrongful injury and may involve litigation. Impairment of sexual function is a recognized injury for which compensation can be claimed regardless of the age and marital status of the victim.
Automobile Plans	Coverage is generally excellent. States with no-fault laws usually establish caps on allowable medical and surgical fees.

Insurance Tips

Insurance companies are typically very happy to receive your premium payments. They are not nearly as enthusiastic when it comes to the payment of claims. In fairness, insurance fraud does exist, and claim examiners must be vigilant to protect the public from ever-rising premium levels. Unfortunately, some claim examiners still do not fully recognize the medical necessity of treatment of male sexual dysfunction, and may be inclined to resist reimbursement of claims in this area.

The following are some useful tips in protecting your personal interests in dealing with insurance companies:

◆ *Fully understand your insurance program.* Read and fully understand the terms and conditions of any existing insurance coverage. If necessary, obtain a complete and detailed description of your coverage. Before making any firm arrangements for treatment, carefully review the "fine print" in your policy. Look especially carefully at sections with titles such as

"not covered," "plan does not pay for," "special limitations," and "exclusions and limitations."

◆ *Be aware of waiting periods.* If changing jobs or
retiring, review your new insurance coverage in advance. Be particularly careful of any waiting periods
that apply to your new coverage or exclusions that
apply to preexisting conditions.

◆ *Obtain prior approval.* Before committing to any treatment program involving a major expenditure, be sure
to obtain prior approval in writing from your insurance
company. Many insurance companies now insist on
prior approval for any type of surgery, and often insist
on a second opinion. Failure to obtain prior approval
can often result in as much as a 50 percent penalty. In
general, obtaining approval requires a demonstration
that the proposed treatment is "medically necessary"
or "reasonable and necessary."

◆ *Use your physician.* Your physician and his or her
professional business staff are a major source of help
on insurance matters. Your physician will play a key
role in obtaining prior approval from your insurance
company, both with respect to communicating your
medical history and explaining the importance of the
treatment from the standpoint of your physical and
mental health and general well-being.

◆ *Recognize the importance of your treatment.* If you
find that you are encountering resistance on the part
of your insurance company, it may be necessary for
you to be insistent in claiming your coverage. Astute
claim examiners are aware that many men subject to
dysfunction may feel awkward and defensive and,
hence, are at a disadvantage. The best way to deal
with this problem is to be fully convinced of the

importance of the treatment to your personal well-being and also to remember that, either directly or indirectly, you paid for the insurance coverage.

FINALLY—A POSSIBLE TAX DEDUCTION

Despite the almost continuous changes that have taken place in the federal income tax law in recent years, significant tax deductions continue to be allowed for legitimate medical and dental expenses, including the cost for treatment of all aspects of male sexual dysfunction. As of 1993, persons who itemize deductions on their federal tax return may take a deduction for all specific categories of medical and dental expense allowable under the tax code. The allowable deduction, however, is limited to that part of total medical and dental expenses in excess of 7.5 percent of "adjusted gross income" as defined and shown on the appropriate line of Form 1040. In general, most states that have an income tax allow a similar deduction.

Expenses in connection with the treatment of sexual dysfunction that are usually deductible include the following:

- The cost of prescription medicine and drugs
- Physicians' professional fees and payments made directly to physicians for tests and drugs
- Payments for tests made directly to medical laboratories
- Psychologist and sex therapist fees
- Hospital costs
- The cost of an implanted penile prosthesis or external vacuum device
- Associated transportation expenses

The various costs incurred in the treatment of sexual dysfunction are, of course, grouped with all other medical and dental expenses on the annual tax return. The expense total can include the annual cost for medical, surgical, and hospitalization insurance. All insurance reimbursement must be subtracted in determining allowable deductible expense.

Given the complexity of the tax code, it is usually advisable to seek advice on tax matters from an accountant or other qualified professional. A possible area of concern as to deductibility could be payments made to psychologists or sex therapists. As it should be clear to the readers of this book, such practitioners should be used judiciously in any event. Another gray area where an accountant could be helpful involves expenses incurred in connection with impotence support groups. These expenses are normally minimal. It is possible that some portion may be treated as a charitable contribution.

It is important to recognize that the overall value of any possible tax deduction for the treatment of sexual dysfunction depends on a variety of factors, including the patient's annual taxable income, the additional income of a spouse, the extent of deductions for other medical and dental services, total deductions of a nonmedical nature, and the amount of insurance coverage. There is no deduction, of course, if deductions are not itemized. In many instances, the indicated 7.5 percent adjusted gross income limitation on medical and dental expenses, combined with good insurance coverage, will effectively cancel out any deduction. On the other hand, the deduction could be of importance, in the case of a patient with a relatively low adjusted gross income, limited insurance coverage, and significant expenditures for medical and dental problems, including treating dysfunction. In addition, there may be other favorable consequences for individuals subject to state and local income taxes.

HELPING YOURSELF THROUGH PREVENTION

In most men, loss of potency is associated with increasing age. The reasons are not difficult to understand. Arteriosclerosis is associated with increasing age. Testosterone production peaks in most men in their thirties. Diabetes often does not appear until well into adulthood. As men age, it becomes more likely that some surgical procedure will be required that could have unfortunate consequences with respect to sexual performance. Also, with increasing age, the ravages of alcohol abuse and tobacco gradually take their toll.

The previous chapters deal with the techniques now available to treat dysfunction problems after they have already made their appearance. This chapter provides some basic tips on what you can do to prevent problems or, at least, to delay their appearance.

223

Men experiencing dysfunction all too often become the marks of quacks and charlatans touting miracle cures. On occasion, some men with perfect sexual function also become victims in the hope of achieving some perceived heroic standard of sexual performance. Impotence fraud has its amusing aspects. The costs, unfortunately, include not only loss of hard-earned cash, but also wasted time and even impairment of health. This chapter provides some basic tips on how to prevent the problems of impotence fraud.

NINE TIPS FOR IMPOTENCE PREVENTION

It has been said that life is sometimes unfair. Even the most responsible individual may suffer from dysfunction as a result of an unavoidable accident or perhaps a military service injury. Genetic factors have been identified in many of the physical conditions linked to impotence. Some men have just been dealt a set of bad genes. Nevertheless, most men do have some options.

The tips for preventing impotence are largely the same as those for maintaining good health: proper nutrition, weight control, reasonable exercise, moderate alcohol consumption, avoidance of tobacco and harmful drugs, and life-style control, including control of sexual activities. It is not our intention to preach on these matters, as most people have already been scolded enough. In fact, there is reason to suspect that constant nagging is actually unproductive. Therefore, the discussions accompanying most of the following tips are mainly limited to brief statements of obvious facts. An exception is the more complicated matter of proper control of your life-style.

Tip 1: Maintain a Proper Diet

Most reasonably well-informed individuals are aware of the general rules for good nutrition. These include controlling the consumption of salt and sodium-containing foods, minimizing total fat intake, avoiding foods high in saturated fats and cholesterol, limiting the intake of refined carbohydrates, and a varied diet that supplies all essential vitamins and minerals. The overall implications are a diet that emphasizes fish, chicken, fruits, vegetables, and whole grains at the expense of red meats, certain dairy products, eggs and junk, fast and processed foods. Properly prepared, such a diet will help to preserve your health, but not with any sacrifice to taste. Appendix E provides some useful dietary suggestions.

Poor diet can result in impotence in three basic ways. First, a diet high in salt and fats can lead to high blood pressure. Unfortunately, as noted, many of the medications used to control hypertension are linked to impotence. Second, a diet high in fats, especially saturated fats and cholesterol, can lead to vascular problems, a major factor underlying impotence. Finally, excessive carbohydrate intake is a factor in diabetes, a major cause of impotence.

Tip 2: Be Sure That Your Diet Provides Certain Vitamins

During the past few years, there has been increased recognition of the importance of antioxidants. Antioxidants are substances that counter the effects of free radicals, highly reactive electrically charged molecules, that will attack any part of the body. Free radicals are constantly produced in the body, as a normal by-product of metabolism, and are essential for many metabolic processes. Oxygen, from the air we breathe, is a key element in free radical formation. Unfortunately, free radicals also are linked to the process of aging and chronic disorders, including heart disease and cancer. Making the situation even worse is the fact that the body can absorb free radicals from tobacco smoke and other environmental pollutants.

Various antioxidants exist, but most current attention is centered on several familiar vitamins with known antioxidant properties: vitamin A, vitamin C, and vitamin E. These vitamins react with and neutralize the free radicals, rendering them harmless.

In the past, there has been a general consensus among nutritionists that a properly balanced diet, in the absence of any nutritional disorder, will normally provide the Recommended Daily Allowance (RDA) for all vitamins and minerals and without any need for vitamin and mineral supplementation. While this is still generally believed, there is an increasing acceptance of the possible value of supplementation in the case of the indicated antioxidant vitamins. The case for supplementation, moreover, is especially compelling, as the body ages or when under conditions of unusual stress.

Vitamin supplements should always be taken with proper precaution. Excess vitamin A in the retinoid form is toxic and can cause liver damage. It is best, therefore, to take beta carotene, a form of vitamin A with far less toxicity. Vitamin C is generally considered nontoxic, but megadoses can cause kidney problems and unpleasant gastritis. Vitamin E is also nontoxic, but excess levels may result in high blood pressure.

Tip 3: Control Your Weight

Good nutrition implies both a properly balanced diet and control of total caloric intake. Obesity contributes directly to both high blood pressure and diabetes. What most people do not know is that there is a natural biochemical conversion of protein to fat, which can take place within the body when caloric intake is excessive. This means that even with a high-protein diet, a possible buildup of fatty substances can result within the vascular system that also contributes to impotence.

Tip 4: Reasonable Exercise

Exercise serves to prevent impotence in several ways. First, a suitable exercise program promotes general cardiovascular fitness. Second, regular exercise lowers blood cholesterol levels. Finally, regular exercise aids considerably in weight control. Sexual activity, incidentally, is a form of exercise, but not one that you can count on for effective weight control. A 5-minute sexual interlude for most men might burn up only 65 calories. Of course, every bit helps.

Most forms of exercise improve cardiovascular fitness. Exceptions are simple calisthenics, weight lifting, and yoga. There is little benefit from golf when golf carts substitute for walking. For most men over 50, regular walking and swimming represent the best bet. Appendix F provides exercise suggestions.

Tip 5: Control Alcohol Consumption

The strong link between alcoholism and impotence was emphasized in Chapter 4. Control of alcohol does not imply total prohibition in an individual not prone to alcoholism. An occasional drink by a nonalcoholic under social circumstances is not a cause for any concern. When consumption begins to regularly exceed two drinks per day, there is good reason to bring things under control.

Good control is also a matter of how fast you drink and what you drink. Drinking slowly puts less strain on the liver, where alcohol is metabolized, and thus serves to minimize long-range adverse effects on testosterone and estrogen levels. Diluted drinks help, as you tend to take in alcohol at a slower rate, and will probably drink less in social circumstances.

Tip 6: Avoid Tobacco

It is difficult to have too much sympathy for any man who is concerned about impotence, but still continues to smoke. Tobacco is one of the most highly addictive substances known, and as such, many men and women are unable to quit even after being diagnosed with tobacco-related disorders such as cancer and heart disease.

The question as to whether secondary tobacco smoke, smoke from the cigarettes of others, can seriously cause adverse consequences, is still a controversial matter. The tobacco industry continues to maintain that secondary smoke is quickly dissipated in the atmosphere. Of course, the tobacco industry still, by and large, refuses to concede that their product is dangerous. Under any circumstances, it would be best to avoid exposure, although obviously this is not always possible. In fact, it is a good idea to attempt to avoid exposure to all airborne pollutants, given their possible cardiovascular consequences. Fortunately, the ban on smoking in domestic air travel now makes it possible to avoid secondary smoke in a situation where particularly high levels of smoke in the past have been common, due to the normal practice of air recirculation.

Tip 7: Avoid Harmful Drugs

The link between impotence and many other controlled substances could be a more compelling reason for some individuals to avoid use than the legal consequences. In the case of legal drugs prescribed by physicians, it is, of course, desirable to avoid use whenever medically possible. The list of drugs linked to impotence, given in Appendix A, should be helpful in this connection. It is a good idea to take the initiative in asking about all possible side effects when obtaining a prescription, and not wait for the physician to volunteer this information.

One area in which you have some control concerns common over-the-counter medications. It is a good idea to avoid most common cold and sleeping remedies, given the possible presence of antihistamines and other chemical entities linked to impotence. Most of these preparations are also of limited effectiveness. When it comes to the relief of cold symptoms, your best bet remains aspirin, acetaminophen, or ibuprofen.

Tip 8: Control Your Life-style

It is conventional wisdom that sexual performance is enhanced by relaxation and the avoidance of stress. While there is some truth to this, it is not always practical. Furthermore, individuals vary greatly in the ways they react to stressful situations.

A letter appearing in *The New York Times* states, "Sexual dysfunction is the first symptom of significant psychopathology in a large percentage of men who are desperately trying to obtain and/or maintain success in the business world." There is a problem with this observation, in that it may give the false impression that impotence is a natural consequence of the stress placed on individuals striving for success. First, there are many highly successful or aspiring men in the business and professional world who continue to perform very well sexually despite crushing day-to-day burdens. Second, there is no hard statistical evidence that business and professional men have a disproportionate incidence of impotence, as compared to men in presumably more bucolic pursuits. Finally, there is considerable evidence that the physical problems associated with impotence—high blood pressure, alcoholism, and so forth—are more common in men at the bottom of the pyramid.

Part of the story could be that it is not so much stress operating through some mysterious pathway of the mind that directly causes impotence, but the longer-range consequence of the way men react to stress. If the only way you can cope with stress is with the three-martini lunch, gorging at the table, or chain smoking, the probability increases that a disease such as arteriosclerosis could, in turn, lead to impotence. If this is the case, a major life-style change involving your job, and probably your income, could represent the only strategy to prevent impotence.

Tip 9: Control Your Sexual Activities

The realities of the aging process suggest reasonable adjustments of past sexual patterns. Sexual activities that take place when the chances for failure are greatest obviously can contribute to performance anxiety. One simple adjustment is to plan for sexual activities first thing in the morning. As testosterone levels are highest in men after a good night's sleep, chances of successful sexual performance are the greatest in these circumstances.

In general, it is a good idea to avoid sexual heroics along with conditions not conducive to sexual performance. The age-old institution of the orgy demonstrates that many men in top physical condition can perform in a highly distracting environment. Most men, however, are stretching their luck under such circumstances. In any event, it is quality that counts in sex, as in every other form of human activity. Also, remember that heroic sex, especially after a period of abstinence, can result in prostate irritation.

HOW TO AVOID BEING "TAKEN"—TIPS FOR IMPOTENCE FRAUD PREVENTION

There is nothing new about impotence fraud. There is good reason, however, to suspect that it is becoming increasingly common. Impotent men, since time immemorial, have been easily taken in because of their especially high degree of vulnerability.

Quacks and charlatans often obtain their victims from responses to advertisements placed in sexually oriented magazines or in magazines with highly macho themes. The ads are typically placed toward the rear of the magazines, accompanied by other ads touting preparations purporting to increase penis size, various devices to be used during sex, "swingers" clubs, and bogus hair growth remedies. Another way that victims are found is through direct mail solicitations. The perpetrators are especially adept at obtaining mailing lists containing the names of older men. Porno stores, such as those found in the vicinity of Times Square in New York City, are another marketing channel.

Quacks with more sophisticated scams, such as pseudoscientific psychotherapy or purported treatments based on the mysteries of the Orient or the occult, sometimes obtain victims through advertisements or through free announcements placed in neighborhood or leisure-time newspapers in large cities. Sometimes, victims are snared through items placed on bulletin boards in health food stores.

The following are a few tips for preventing impotence fraud:

Tip 1: Beware of All Solicitations That Use a Blatantly Suggestive Sexual Theme

Solicitations that contain soft-porn pictures or titillating advertising copy deserve to be rejected. Impotence is a medical problem, and while promotional activities are permitted to some extent in the medical field, such activities are limited to the presentation of factual material and generally accepted standards of good taste.

*Tip 2: Beware of All Solicitations That Are Too Good to Be True or
      That Are Ridiculous*

Fraud should be suspected whenever a solicitation offers to provide a medication, service, or some form of information that offers rapid and guaranteed results. The only
medications now in common use for treatment of impotence
have been discussed in Chapter 7 and are further listed in
Appendix D. All these drugs should be used only under
medical supervision. Nevertheless, the African rhinoceros
has become an endangered species due to the continuing
belief in the Far East that the ground horn of a rhinoceros will
improve potency. Young men continue to be taken in Tijuana
and other border cities by the hawkers of "Spanish fly."

Some forms of medication promoted by quacks can be
dangerous. One example is chelation therapy, which has
been promoted for treatment of hardening of the arteries, as
well as for impotence. Men sometimes sniff amyl nitrate and
other aromatic substances in the belief that it enhances the
orgasm. The real result may be a severe headache or even
damage to internal organs.

Penis size nostrums are often sold with ridiculous
claims that promise not only a dramatic increase in physical
dimensions, but also an extraordinary improvement in the
buyer's sexual fortunes. Surgical enhancement of penile
girth and length, as discussed in Chapter 10, is the only
known means of altering the size of the visible penis.

*Tip 3: Beware of All Solicitations from Individuals with Question-
      able Professional Qualifications*

It is a mistake to believe that the medical establishment
is the repository of all wisdom. The history of medicine does
include many instances of the rejection of ideas later proven
to be valid. Outsiders, such as the chemist Louis Pasteur,
have also made major contributions to the medical field.

Nevertheless, there is very good reason to be cautious of solicitations made by individuals with credentials well out of the mainstream or with no credentials at all, or of solicitations by misunderstood or rejected would-be geniuses.

A few excerpts from a direct mail solicitation bearing a North Carolina return address sum it all up:

Close your eyes and imagine the ecstasy of making love to a woman like the one whose picture is enclosed. [The solicitation includes a glossy, 3- by 5-inch color photograph of an attractive, suggestively clad woman].

If you're not as firm as you were in your teens and 20s—let me tell you about a natural way to regain rock solid potency that works like a miracle.

After years of frustration, I met an old friend. He told me how his sex life had turned around by following some very simple instructions.

The secrets that my friend revealed to me have been published in a special report: "How to Restore Your Potency." And now for the good news. "How to Restore Your Potency" is yours for only $19.95.

"How to Restore Your Potency" will do just that—restore your potency. If it does not, you may return the report for double your money back.

Thinking that perhaps we had missed something, we rushed off our $19.95 payment. About a week later, a 21-page soft-cover booklet arrived in the mail. The secret promised in the advertisement turned out to be "Shiatsu," a method of massage described as "the ancient Oriental technique for erotic arousal." Shiatsu is said to be widely practiced in Turkey, Egypt, China, and Japan and obviously for good reason. Shiatsu will not only restore your potency, but will cure chronic constipation, skin rash, headaches, backaches, ulcers, and even heart conditions.

How to perform Shiatsu is described at length in the booklet, including such valuable details as proper room temperature; the use of banana, almond, and avocado oils; and the suggestions that nails should be trimmed very short to avoid scratching. Among the more fascinating items of extraneous information provided is the revelation that men who prefer women with small buttocks generally were breast fed as infants and do not read sports magazines. Women with large buttocks, however, are valued by men who, among other things, are orderly in their everyday affairs.

Don't say that you weren't warned.

CHAPTER 13

A MESSAGE TO THE PARTNER

Struggling with the burden of male sexual dysfunction is more than just a problem faced by the afflicted man. The impact on you, the partner, can be equally as devastating. Furthermore, you may already suspect that other members of your family unit sense something is very wrong.

With impotence, the female partner and any other members of the household bear the burden of day-to-day living with a deeply troubled man. This is a man who questions his very self-worth. The internal torment comes out in different ways, depending on the man. Perhaps your partner is the type of man who keeps it all to himself. He never talks about the subject and deliberately avoids the tender moments you once so much enjoyed out of fear that it could lead to still another sexual disappointment. Then again, your partner could be the type who frets incessantly over the problem. He repeatedly attempts intercourse, each time becoming more visibly discouraged.

No matter how he handles the problem, you are increasingly alarmed about certain aspects of his behavior. He always used to be so easy to get along with. Now he seems to snap at you every time you talk to him. His views about almost everything are tinged with bitterness. He is drinking much more heavily and, after many years of abstinence, has resumed smoking. He is having problems on the job. He is obviously deeply depressed and has said several times recently that life is hardly worth living.

You, of course, have your own sexual needs, but you are afraid to say anything. Perhaps you consider your sexual drive relatively modest and are willing to accept lack of fulfillment. Nevertheless, the problem has filled you with self-doubts and perhaps even suspicions. Maybe it is something that you have or have not done. Maybe he no longer considers your physical appearance attractive. Maybe he no longer considers you interesting to be with. Perhaps his problem has been caused by your lack of enthusiasm or imagination when you make love. Then again, perhaps the real problem is that your partner is having an affair, leaving him too worn out for sex with you at home.

Perhaps you are of the age to have children and want to do so. How can this ever be possible given your partner's problem? Maybe having children is not such a good idea, anyway, given the way things have been going.

Unfortunately, there are no miracle solutions. The following, however, are a few tips that could be helpful:

Tip 1: Tell Your Partner That You Fully Realize a Serious Problem Exists

When an impotence episode occurs, it is a very common pattern for women to attempt to console their partners with statements such as, "It's not important" or "It doesn't matter." Such words, while sincere and loving in intent, are often very counterproductive. Despite what is being said, the man knows that the problem really does matter, and not only to himself.

It is far better to tell your partner that you know there is a serious problem that very much matters to both of you. Emphasize to your partner that you know the problem is not due to any failing on his part. Make it clear that you know there are effective solutions. Finally, tell him that this is something that both of you are going to work out together.

Tip 2: Encourage Your Partner to Perform the Personal Evaluation Outlined in Chapter 5

The personal evaluation outlined in Chapter 5 should help you decide whether the problem could be just temporary or something that requires immediate professional attention. Assist your partner whenever possible in making the evaluation. Make a game that both of you can play out of the simple physical tests given in the chapter.

A little humor in the situation, even gallows humor, should help both of you. Moreover, you may find that just the fact you are doing something together will make both of you feel much better.

Tip 3: If Indicated, Encourage Your Partner to Seek Prompt Professional Attention

If the personal evaluation suggests the problem is more than temporary, encourage your partner to immediately seek professional attention. Be especially insistent whenever there is reason to suspect that the impotence problem could be the result of a serious underlying physical problem, such as diabetes. It is also important to let your partner know that the logical way to deal with impotence is to first investigate the possibility of a physical cause. Encourage him to review the material on where to get help in Chapter 6.

Tip 4: Become Personally Familiar with the Causes of Impotence or Any Other Dysfunction Problem That Your Partner May Be Experiencing

While there is no need to become an expert on the subject, it will be potentially very helpful for both of you if you become familiar with the various conditions that can underlie impotence. It can be surprisingly comforting to know that impotence can often have a physical, rather than a psychological, cause. This helps to alleviate any guilt feelings that you or your partner may be experiencing. It also makes you an active partner in the solution of the problem.

Tip 5: Become Personally Familiar with Treatment Methods

The more you know about treatment methods, the better position you will be in to assist your partner whenever an important decision as to treatment is required. It is particularly important that you share all decisions regarding a possible penile implant. Also, the more familiar you become with treatment methods, the more helpful you will be to your partner during the actual treatment program.

Tip 6: Participate, Whenever Appropriate, in the Treatment Program

Take advantage of every opportunity to participate in the treatment program. One way you might possibly help would be to keep a chronological record of your partner's physical response at various stages of the program. Your urologist may ask you to accompany your partner on office visits to provide your insights.

Tip 7: Help Your Partner Improve His Life-style

It is never too late to adopt a healthy life-style more compatible with successful sexual performance. If your partner smokes, for example, help him to quit. One way to help greatly would be to quit yourself, if you are a smoker. Similar advice applies to moderating alcohol consumption and eating a healthy diet.

Tip 8: Investigate Alternative Sexual Techniques

Investigate possible ways for you and your partner to achieve mutual sexual satisfaction that do not require full vaginal penetration. It is important to let your partner understand that you do not consider this a substitute for the "real thing," but rather something you can do temporarily while the two of you work together to overcome the impotence problem.

Tip 9: Don't Give Up If You Want to Have Children

If having children is a factor, it is important that you personally recognize that as long as your partner can ejaculate by masturbation, you can have children. The process would not be much different than would be the case with artificial insemination, and the baby will be just as precious. Be sure that your partner is aware of these facts.

Tip 10: Consider Joining a Support Group with Your Partner

Participation in an impotence support group can prove to be very helpful. Such groups will provide you with valuable information relevant to your problem. Contact with persons with similar problems could prove comforting, as you learn that your problems are not unique and that others have achieved effective solutions.

Workable treatments now exist for male sexual dysfunction. The treatments, of course, are not perfect. After all, there is still no way to repair destroyed nerves or to flush accumulated plaque out of arteries. Available techniques, such as the implant, however, have been found to be very effective.

It is certain that great strides in treatment will occur over the next few years. Remember that only little more than a decade ago, there was very little hope for many patients. Even true psychological impotence can be expected to yield to convenient and economical treatment in the future.

Finally, be aware that solving a male sexual dysfunction problem is not a cure-all for a badly flawed relationship. Working together with your partner to solve the problem, however, can actually strengthen a basically sound relationship. That is what Susan and Jesse, whom you met at the beginning of the book, found out.

SOME QUESTIONS PATIENTS ASK

Whenever you visit a physician for any medical problem, never hesitate to ask questions. The following are some of the questions that our patients have asked:

My internist says that impotence is largely a matter of age. Does this mean that impotence is inevitable as you grow older?

Comment: Your internist's observation has an element of truth, but it is misleading. There is little question that if you take a large group of men at random, there will be a higher incidence of erectile failure among the older men in the group. This does not mean that age, in itself, is the cause of impotence or that impotence is an inevitable consequence of the aging process. The explanation is with the passage of time the chances are that you will experience one or more of the disorders or traumas that can cause impotence such as cardiovascular disease, diabetes, or pelvic injury. If you are fortunate enough not to experience any such problem, it is entirely possible that you will be able to maintain sexual function throughout your lifetime.

Is there any truth to the idea that impotence is inherited?

Comment: It is a fact that in recent years, an increasing number of medical disorders have been shown to have a genetic link. In many cases, specific genes underlying various disorders have been identified. Given the general neglect of the problem of erectile dysfunction until recent years, however, it is not surprising that there has yet to be any real study of whether impotence can run in families. It is not unreasonable to suspect that the penile vascular structure and nerve connections of some men place them at greater risk of erectile dysfunction at some point during their lives than others and that such characteristics could be inherited. There is also evidence that genetics plays a role in cardiovascular disease and cardiovascular disease, of course, is a factor in impotence. It would be fortunate if someday medical science identifies an impotence gene, leading to the possibility of treating impotence with gene therapy.

I have heard of something called the male menopause. Can there be any connection with impotence?

Comment: The word "menopause" usually refers to that stage of a women's life characterized by the cessation of monthly menstrual periods and the loss of fertility. The female menopause also corresponds to time in a women's life when there is a significant fall in the production of the principal female sex hormone, estrogen. It has been suggested by some observers that something similar can occur in men associated possibly with a decline in testosterone production. Some observers have used the word "viropause," instead of male menopause, thus suggesting a connection with diminished sexual virility.

Obviously, if there is a male menopause, nothing noticeable takes place comparable to the ending of monthly periods. In addition, many men continue to produce sperm and are able to father children throughout life. Testosterone production, however, does slowly decline in middle age. It is also true that many men experience so-called middle-life crises, characterized by anger, withdrawal, and depression.

At this time, there is no conclusive evidence proving that the male menopause really exists in a physical sense. It is also reasonable to suspect that many of the symptoms associated with middle-life crises are psychological, resulting from diminished career expectations, family conflict, and so forth or are due to the emotional consequences of physical impotence caused not by male menopause, but rather by such tangible factors as cardiovascular disease. Nevertheless, it is also true that certain men with erectile dysfunction exhibit abnormally low testosterone levels and can sometimes be helped by testosterone injections.

I'm 47 and married, but I still frequently masturbate. Can this in anyway affect my sexual performance?

Comment: First, it should be recognized that masturbation is very common among partners in stable relationships. Some studies have indicated that roughly 70 percent of both men and women in stable relationships will masturbate on a fairly regular basis. There is no evidence that masturbation will affect the sexual performance of men in any negative manner. Of course, when a man masturbates to ejaculation, the usual refractory or recovery period will have to take place before intercourse can be attempted.

Some recent, fascinating findings from research conducted at the University of Manchester in the United Kingdom suggest that masturbation may have evolved as a means of enhancing male fertility. According to these studies, aging sperm are characterized by lower energy levels, deformed tails, and reduced swimming capabilities. When a man first ejaculates after a period of abstinence, the most aged sperm present in the body departs first and such sperm is least likely to accomplish fertilization. The University of Manchester study also reveals that more than half of the time normal sexual intercourse will take place within 48 hours following masturbation. In other words, masturbation may serve the purpose of clearing out aged sperm and making sure that the sperm discharged during intercourse is of the highest quality suitable for the propagation of the species.

What is the connection between prostate problems and impotence?

Comment: The prostate plays an important, but still not fully understood, role in male sexuality. The prostate has been called the gland that always goes wrong, indicating that, sooner or later, almost every man will experience some form of prostate problem. It is known that prostate infections can be a factor in causing premature ejaculation. There is no real evidence, however, that prostate infections can cause impotence, although men with prostate infections may experience pain and discomfort when engaging in sexual intercourse and may avoid intercourse for this reason.

The presence of a prostate tumor, either benign or malignant, in itself will not usually cause impotence. In some cases, removal of the prostate gland is not followed by impotence, indicating that the gland, by itself, is not essential for erection to take place. It is true, however, that treatment of such tumors by surgery, radiation, or hormonal therapy will very often result indirectly in impotence as an unavoidable side effect.

> *I find that I have an increasing problem obtaining an erection without penile manipulation. Recently, I was with a women who was reluctant to manipulate my penis and became upset when I manipulated myself. Should I be able to obtain an erection by merely being in an erotic situation?*

Comment: In young men, involuntary erections often take place merely in casual conversation with particularly desirable young women. As we grow older, this experience becomes still another wistful memory of days gone by. In general, as men age it requires an increasing degree of physical stimulation of the penis to achieve an erection satisfactory for intercourse. This, by no means necessarily, implies that erectile dysfunction exists or that can be anticipated to occur in the near future.

The female partner often provides the necessary physical stimulation of the penis during the foreplay period prior to intercourse. It is not at all unusual or wrong for a man to provide the manipulation himself. When a women objects to providing manipulation, it may indicate a general aversion to sex or the somewhat vain belief that her physical presence alone should be sufficient to raise an erection. When a women objects to the man providing self-manipulation, it could be indicative of a negative attitude toward masturbation based on religious and cultural values.

> *Is there any connection between cancer and impotence?*

Comment: In general, cancer is not regarded as an important cause of impotence. Cancer, or uncontrolled cell growth, often affects various parts of the body by crowding out normal tissue and interfering with essential metabolic processes. When the point of attack is any of the glands that produce male sexual hormones, the result can be loss of desire and erectile dysfunction. Cancer can also result in impotence indirectly as when prostate cancer necessitates surgery, radiation therapy, or hormonal treatment.

I'm considering having a vasectomy. Could this lead to any type of sexual dysfunction?

Comment: There is no convincing evidence of a physical link between impotence and vasectomy. A relatively small number of men who have had a vasectomy react emotionally, and in some instances, this can lead to performance difficulties of a psychological nature. A factor often present in such cases is the mistaken belief that infertility and impotence are somehow connected. Such men may reason that an infertile man is somehow something less than a full male and hence incapable of erection, as well as having children. Urologists attempt to screen out such men before performing the vasectomy procedure.

It should be pointed out that one recent study suggests a possible link between vasectomy and prostate cancer. This study is yet to be confirmed, and in any event, the increased risk is not especially alarming. If you are considering having a vasectomy, you should discuss this matter with your urologist.

I have heard that saltpeter prevents a man from having an erection. It is not included among the drugs listed in this book as being linked to impotence. Can saltpeter cause a problem?

Comment: Saltpeter is a inorganic nitrate substance. Just plain saltpeter is potassium nitrate. Sodium nitrate is known as Chile saltpeter, reflecting the fact that much of the world supply of that chemical comes from Chile. Saltpeter has many uses, but the only time it normally gets ingested by the body is when it is used for pickling meat.

There is a common belief that eating meats prepared with saltpeter will result in temporary loss of erectile function. A popular myth is that large quantities of such meat are served at teenage boy's camps, to discourage masturbation. There is no evidence that eating an occasional, delicious New York–style corned beef or pastrami sandwich or corned beef and cabbage on St. Patrick's Day is a sure way not to have an erection. If there were, saltpeter might have been investigated as a means of preventing unwanted erections during certain urological surgical procedures. It is a good idea, incidentally, to limit your consumption of meats prepared with saltpeter, as such products are often fatty and nitrates, in general, are suspect in connection with cancer.

I have heard that men who have been circumcised experience less sexual sensation. Can this result in impotence?

Comment: It is true that removal of the foreskin does result in some minor loss of sexual sensation in the glans, or forward head of the penis. There is no evidence that this is sufficient to cause erectile dysfunction. In this connection, it is worth noting that multiple wives are common in many Islamic countries where circumcision is practiced due to religious belief. Many such countries are also characterized by explosive population growth.

It seems as if it takes my partner forever to achieve an orgasm. I very often either lose my erection or ejaculate too soon. Does this mean that I have a dysfunction problem?

Comment: No, it does not follow that you have an erectile dysfunction problem. Some women are incapable of ever experiencing orgasm during conventional sexual intercourse no matter how long the male partner is able to sustain an erection. Under these circumstances, the man should assist his partner by other means.

> *I find that I get a fully satisfactory erection most of the time. Sometimes I get only a partial erection or an erection that is lost very rapidly. What is going on?*

Comment: Such symptoms are fairly typical of a developing erectile dysfunction problem. They can be the result of some ongoing life-style problem. Under the circumstances, you should keep an accurate chronological record indicating the dates and time of day that you have attempted intercourse, the prevailing conditions (including such factors as privacy, whether you have been drinking, and the attitude of your partner), and your resulting sexual performance. If conditions appear to worsen over a period of time, it would be a good idea to see a urologist. You should also try the various tests discussed in Chapter 5.

> *The information provided in this book on where to seek treatment for male sexual dysfunction is largely directed toward the American reader. Is treatment available outside the United States and is there any advantage in seeking such treatment?*

Comment: Although the United States has been a leader in the treatment of male sexual dysfunction, excellent work has been underway in many of the countries of the European Community and Japan. There is also very good work being done in neighboring Canada. In general, Europeans have placed greater emphasis in the past on reconstructive surgery than Americans, but differences in treatment approaches have been disappearing as more is learned about male sexual dysfunction and cooperation among urologists throughout the world becomes commonplace. Unfortunately, no where in the world are there any magic cures. Under the circumstances, there is very little reason for an American to seek overseas treatment.

Impotence is a sensitive subject and still often misunderstood. Will my privacy be protected if I seek treatment?

Comment: It is indeed a sensitive subject and one that is still very much misunderstood. Despite the willingness of some persons to tell all on talk shows, many men have good reason to prevent their problem from being known by casual friends and employers. Men in public life have very special reasons for demanding privacy.

When you bring your problem to a urologist, you can expect your condition to be kept confidential due to traditional standards of medical ethics. In this connection, all the cases discussed in this book have been carefully disguised in order to protect the patients. The area of insurance reimbursement, however, can present a problem. Information required for insurance claims is now stored in a computerized data base as a matter of routine. The chances of any such information getting into the hands of the wrong individuals and causing embarrassment are small, and there is increasing public awareness of the need for effective measures to guard the confidentiality of medical records.

This book discusses a wide variety of treatment alternatives. How does a urologist arrive at the best treatment choice for every individual patient?

Comment: The process by which physicians arrive at the best treatment for any medical problem is known as "staging." In treating erectile dysfunction, the logical first stage is to determine whether the problem has a physical cause or is psychological. When the latter, the patient may be referred to a psychotherapist or a sex therapist. When a physical cause can be identified, the usual approach is to consider the least invasive, with minimal side effects, possible. This can possibly involve switching to an alternate drug if a drug currently being used to treat high blood pressure is suspect, trying testosterone injections when abnormally low levels of testosterone are detected, trying a drug such as yohimbine, or using an external vacuum device. Subsequent stages would include penile injection therapy or installation of a penile implant. In general, vascular surgery would not be undertaken except in special cases. Of course, some of the intermediate stages noted may be skipped when the most effective treatment is obvious under the circumstances.

Can exercise reverse impotence?

Comment: Exercise should be largely regarded as a means of prevention. Unfortunately, it has only minimal effect on restoring damaged portions of the vascular system involved in the erectile process. Exercise, combined with weight control, may in some instances control high blood pressure and eliminate the need to take a drug linked to impotence. In such a case, it may be reasoned that exercise has played a role in reversing impotence. There are also reports that Kegel exercises, discussed in Appendix F, can have some positive effect on sexual performance.

Still on the subject of exercise, is there any truth to the belief that when a man has sex prior to athletic competition his performance will suffer?

Comment: This is an age-old myth, without any scientific foundation, that nevertheless is widely believed. It is partially based on an ancient belief that the semen somehow represents some kind of vital force that serves as the basis of a man's strength. Also underlying the myth is the sexist belief that women wish to drain men of their power. Actually, a healthy pattern of sex should serve to enhance the performance of both men and women in athletics, as well as other activities.

> *What is the connection between zinc and male sexual dysfunction?*

Comment: The belief that taking supplements of zinc will improve erectile function stems from the fact that the mineral is present in the prostate gland at a very high level of concentration. The prostate gland, of course, is associated in many minds with male sexuality. The reason for the presence of zinc is, at present, not fully understood. One explanation that has been suggested is that zinc has some positive effect on the health of the sperm and thus serves to promote fertility. No link has been established in the processes that control erection. Therefore, there is little reason to hope that taking zinc supplements will cure an erectile dysfunction problem.

> *I have heard that eating raw pumpkin seeds, peanuts, and pecans can help male sexual performance. Is there anything to this?*

Comment: Pumpkin seeds, peanuts, and pecans are tasty foods that do contain valuable vitamins and minerals. These vitamins and minerals, however, are all obtainable from other food sources. Pumpkin seeds, which do contain a unique nonvolatile oil, do have a medical use in the treatment of intestinal worms. There have been claims that large colonies of worms in the lower bowel can cause prostate enlargement. This tenuous link to the prostate has probably been a factor in fostering the belief that raw pumpkin seeds can help erectile dysfunction. There also have been unsubstantiated claims that pumpkin seeds contain a natural male hormone. Unless you have a very specific allergy, there is no reason not to eat reasonable quantities of pumpkin seeds, peanuts, and pecans in the hope that it might do some good. Unfortunately, no magic substance is yet to be found in any type of food that will cure erectile dysfunction.

DRUGS THAT MAY CAUSE MALE SEXUAL DYSFUNCTION

The following is a listing of drugs by generic and brand names that have been linked in various reports to erectile failure and several other male sexual dysfunction problems. Note that some brand-name drugs appear more than once on list due to the presence of more than one active generic ingredient in its formulation.

Should you be taking any drug shown and are currently experiencing dysfunction, it does not necessarily follow that the drug is the root cause of your problem. Another and more important underlying factor may be at work. It is also important to recognize that often a drug has been implicated in a published report, based on anecdotal evidence alone and in the absence of a systematic research study of its sexual side effects. In addition, you should be aware that all men do not

253

react in the same manner when taking any given drug. Should you be simultaneously taking more than one of the drugs shown, or one of the drugs along with some unlisted medication, the possibility exists that the combination of drugs could result in enhanced side effects. You should also be aware that cigarette smoking has been shown to exacerbate the dysfunction problems associated with many of the drugs shown.

If you are taking any of the drugs listed here and are experiencing a dysfunction problem, bring this fact promptly to the attention of your physician.. Your physician may be able to prescribe alternate medication. If possible, keep a log indicating the times you took the suspected medication and the time you experienced sexual problems. Under no circumstance should you discontinue use of any prescription on your own, as this could result in serious health consequences.

Additional information on the sexual side effects of prescription drugs can be obtained from the *Physician's Desk Reference* (Oradell, NJ: Medical Economics Company, annually). This comprehensive reference book can be found at most larger public libraries or at your physician's office. A companion volume by the same publisher, *The Physician's Desk Refernce for Nonprescription Drugs*, provides information on the side effects of over-the-counter producys. For information on the side effects of drugs used for controlling the emotions, a useful resource is Stuart Yudof, M.D., et al., *What You Need to Know About Psychiatric Drugs* (New York: Grove Weldenfeld, 1991.).

DRUGS LINKED TO IMPOTENCE

Cardiovascular Drugs (for High Blood Pressure, Heart Disease, Cholesterol Control, and Related Problems)

Generic (Technical) Name	*Brand Name(s)*
Chlorthalidone	Combipres Demi-Regroton Hygroton
Chlorothiazide	Diuril
Clofibrate	Altromid-S
Clonidine hydrochloride	Catapres, Combipres
Digitalis	Crystodigen
Digoxin	Lanoxicaps, Lanoxin
Disopyramide phosphate	Norpace
Guanethidine sulfate	Esmil, Ismelin
Hydrochlorothiazide	Aldactazide, Aldoril, Apesazide, Dyazide, Esidrix, Esimil, HydroDiuril, Hydropres, Inderide, Moduretic tablets, Ser-Ap-Es
Metoprolol	Lopressor
Methylodopa	Aldoclor, Aldomet, Aldoril
Pargyline hydrochloride	Eutonyl, Eutron
Phenoxybenzamine hydrochloride	Dibenzyline
Phentolamine	Regitine
Propranolol	Inderal, Inderide
Rauwolfia serpentina	Harmonyl, Raudixin, Rauzide tablets

Reserpine   Demi-Regroton Diupres,
                                       Hydropres, Metatesin,
                                       Regroton, Salutesin,
                                       Sandril, Ser-Ap-Es,
                                       Serpasil

Spironolactone   Aldactazine, Aldactone

Drugs for Controlling the Emotions (Tranquilizers, Antidepressants, Antianxiety Agents)

Generic (Technical) Name   *Brand Name(s)*

Amitriptyline   Elavil, Endep, Etrafon,
                                       Limbitrol, Triavil

Chlordiazepoxide   Librium, Limbitrol,
                                       Menrium

Chlorpromazine   Thorazine

Chlorprothizine   Taractan

Clomipramine hydrochloride   Anafranil

Clorazepate dipotassium   Tranxene

Desipramine   Norpramin, Pertofrane

Diazepam   Valium, Valrelease
                                       capsules

Droperidol   Inapsine, Innovar

Fluphenazine   Permitil, Prolixin

Haloperidol   Haldon

Imipramine   Janimine, Tofranil

Isocarboxazide   Marplan

Lithium carbonate   Eslalith, Lithane, lithobid,
                                       Lithonate, Lithotabs

Maprotiline hydrochloride   Ludiomil

Mesoridazine   Serentil

Meprobamate	Deprol, Equanil, Equagesic, Meprospan, Milpath, Miltown
Nortriptyline	Aventyl, Pamelor
Oxazepam	Serax
Pargylene	Eutonyl
Phenelzine sulfate	Nardil
Procarbazine hydrochloride	Matulane
Protriptyline hydrochloride	Vivactil
Prochloperazine	Combid, Compazine, Prochlor-Iso
Promazine	Sparine
Trifluroperazine	Stelazine
Trimipramine maleate	Surmontil
Thioridazine	Mellaril
Thiothixene	Navane
Tranicypromine sulfate	Parnate
Tybamate	Tybatran

Antihistamines (Treatment of Allergies, Common Cold Preparations, Sleeping Pills, and Motion Sickness Remedies)

Generic (Technical) Name	*Brand Name(s)*
Dimenhydrinate	Dramamine, Nico-Vert
Diphenhydramine	Ambenyl, Benadryl, Benylin, Bromanyl, Dytuss
Hydroxzine	Vistaril
Meclizine	Antivert, Bonine

Promethazine

Dihydrocodeine Compound
Maxigesic, Mepergan
Phenergan, Remsed,
Stopayne, Synalgos,
Zipan

Drugs for Gastrointestinal Problems (Ulcers, Heartburn, Stomach Pain, Flatulence, and Spastic Colon and Bowels)

Generic (Technical) Name	*Brand Name(s)*
Atropine	Antrocol, Arco-Lase Pills, Butabell, Probocon, Uretron
Propantheline bromide	Pro-Banthine
Cimetidine	Tagamet
Metoclopramide	Regian
Ranitidine hydrochloride	Zantac

Drugs Used for Treating Benign and Malignant Prostate Tumors

Generic (Technical) Name	*Brand Name(s)*
Estradiol (estrogen)	Estrace
Finasteride	Proscar
Flutamine	Eulexin
Gosereline acetate	Zoladex
Leuprolide acetate	Lupron

Drugs Used for Other Medical Problems[1]

Generic (Technical) Name	*Brand Name(s)*
Accteozolamide (glaucoma)	Diamox
Aminocaproic acid (bleeding)	Amicar
Benztropine (Parkinson's disease)	Cogentin
Biperidin (Parkinson's disease)	Akineton
Cycrimine (Parkinson's disease)	Pagitane
Cyclybenzaprine (muscle spasms)	Flexeril
Disulfiram (alchoholism)	Antabuse
Ethionamide (tuberculosis)	Trecator-SC
Indomethacin (arthritis)	Indocin
Methysergide (severe headaches)	Sansert
Metronidzole (infections)	Flagyl, Satric
Trihexyphenidyl (Parkinson's disease)	Artane
Orphenadrine (muscle spasms)	Norflex, Norgesic, X-Otag
Phenytoin (grand mal seizures)	Dilantin
Procyclidine (Parkinson's disease)	Kemadrin

1 Principal medical use of drug in parentheses.

Drugs Linked to Ejaculatory Failure[2]

Generic (Technical) Name	*Brand Name(s)*
Chlorpromazine (emotional control)	Thorazine
Clomipramine (emotional control)	Anafranil
Clonidine hydrochloride (cardiovascular problems)	Catapres, Combipres
Estradiol (prostate tumors)	Estrace
Guanethidine sulfate (cardovascular problems)	Esimil, Ismelin
Methylodopa (cardiovascular problems)	Aldomet
Phenoxybenzamine hydrochloride (controlling emotions)	Dibenzyline
Reserpine (cardiovascular problems)	Demi-Regroton, Diupres, Hydropres, Metatesin, Regroton, Salutesin, Sandril, Ser-Ap-Es, Serpasil
Thioridazine (emotional control)	Mellaril

Drugs Linked to Priapism[3]

Generic (Technical) Name	*Brand Name(s)*
Chloropromazine (emotional control)	Thorazine

2 Principal medical use of drug in parentheses.
3 Principal medical use of drug in parentheses.

Levodopa (Parkinson's disease)	Dopar
Thioridazine (emotional control)	Mellaril
Trazodone (emotional problems)	Desyrel

Drugs Linked to Retrograde Ejaculation[4]

Generic (Technical) Name   *Brand Name*

Thioridazine (emotional control)   Mellaril

Drugs Linked to Loss of Sexual Desire (Libido)[5]

Generic (Technical) Name	*Brand Name(s)*
Amitriptyline (emotional control)	Elavil, Endep, Etrafon, Limbitrol, Triavil
Amoxapine (emotional control)	Asendin
Chlordiazepoxide (emotional control)	Librium, Limbitrol, Menrium
Chloropromazine (emotional control)	Thorazine
Cimetidine (gastrointestinal problems)	Tagamet
Clomipramine hydrochloride (emotional control)	Anafranil

4 Principal medical use of drug in parentheses.
5 Principal medical use of drug in parentheses.

Clonidine hydrochloride (cardiovascular problems)	Catapres, Combipres
Despiramine (emotional control)	Norpramin, Pertofrane
Diazepam (emotional control)	Valium, Valrelease capsules
Disulfiram (alcoholism)	Antabuse
Doxepin hydrochloride (emotional control)	Adalpin, Sinequan
Estradiol (prostate tumors)	Estrace
Flutamine (prostate tumors)	Eulexin
Imipramine (emotional control)	Hanimine, Tofranil
Leuprolide acetate (prostate tumors)	Lupron
Maprotiline hydrochloride (emotional control)	Ludiomil
Methydopa (cardiovascular problems)	Aldomet
Nortiplyline (emotional control)	Aventyl, Pamelor
Protriptyline hydrochloride (emotional control)	Vivactil
Ranitidine hydrochloride (gastrointestinal problems)	Zantac
Reserpine (cardiovascular problems)	Demi-Regroton, Diupres, Hydropres, Metatesin, Regroton, Salutesin, Sandril, Ser-Ap-Es, Serpasil
Tripramine maleate (emotional control)	Surmontil

SAMPLE MEDICAL HISTORY QUESTIONNAIRE

All new patients at the Morganstern Urology Clinic, P.C., Atlanta, Georgia, are requested to complete the medical history questionnaire that follows. You will assist your physician and yourself by carefully compiling the indicated information prior to your initial visit for treatment of any sexual dysfunction problem. The form shown in this appendix may differ, of course, from that used by your own physician, but it does include most questions that may be asked.

Dear Patient:

This is a "preliminary history" and, as is the case of all medical records, is confidential. I will go over the pertinent points with you, and you can make explanations, ask questions, and give any additional information. Your completing this form in advance will give me a more detailed and accurate appraisal of your problem. It is understood that memory and recall of past medical events is not always complete or precise, but please answer each question carefully and to the best of your ability. Do not worry about questions you cannot answer or do not understand; leave these questions unanswered for the present. If this has been mailed to you, please bring it with you for your first visit.

Thank you,

Steven L. Morganstern, M. D.

Patient's Name _____ **Date** _____

Present Illness or Problem

1. Please state the reason or symptom that brought you to a urologist _____

_____

_____

_____

2. How long has the illness or problem existed? _____

_____

Past or ongoing Urological Problems

Please answer as to whether you have had in the past, or now have a problem relating to any of the following (check yes or no):

	Yes	No (If Needed)	Date and Comment
1. Passage of stones or "gravel"	[ ]	[ ]	_____
2. Blood in the urine	[ ]	[ ]	_____
3. Burning on urination	[ ]	[ ]	_____
4. Frequency of urination by day	[ ]	[ ]	_____
5. Getting up at night to urinate (number of times)	[ ]	[ ]	_____
6. Unusually small size of urinary stream	[ ]	[ ]	_____
7. Hesitation of urination prior to starting to void	[ ]	[ ]	_____
8. A weak urinary stream	[ ]	[ ]	_____
9. Straining to urinate	[ ]	[ ]	_____
10. Stopping and starting while urinating	[ ]	[ ]	_____
11. Pain with intercourse	[ ]	[ ]	_____
12. Pain over the bladder region	[ ]	[ ]	_____

13. Pain over the kidney region	[ ] [ ]	_____
14. Fevers of undetermined cause	[ ] [ ]	_____
15. Kidney or bladder infections	[ ] [ ]	_____
16. Other kidney disease	[ ] [ ]	_____
17. Prostatic or testicular disease	[ ] [ ]	_____
18. Urinary incontinence (accidentally losing urine)	[ ] [ ]	_____
19. Childhood bedwetting At what age did you stop bedwetting?	[ ] [ ]	_____
20. Urethral stricture	[ ] [ ]	_____
21. Previous kidney X rays (I.V.P.)	[ ] [ ]	_____
22. Previous cystoscopic exam	[ ] [ ]	_____
23. Previous urologic surgery	[ ] [ ]	_____

24. How many times usually, on average, do you void each day _____ each night _____

25. Any other problems you have had that may relate to your genital or urinary system including the following:

a. Impotence (erectile failure)	[ ] [ ]	_____
b. Premature ejaculation	[ ] [ ]	_____
c. Failure to ejaculate	[ ] [ ]	_____
d. Priapism (an unwanted erection)	[ ] [ ]	_____
e. Lack of sexual desire	[ ] [ ]	_____
f. Penis deformed when erect	[ ] [ ]	_____
g. Infertility	[ ] [ ]	_____
h. Fear of sex	[ ] [ ]	_____

i. Other _____

_____

_____

General Medical History

Have you had any of the illnesses listed below? Please place a check in the appropriate column. If you are reasonably certain that you have had, or now have, a given disease or disorder, indicate either your age or the year when the illness occurred, or first developed, in the "Age or Date" column. Age periods such as infancy, child-hood, or teens are acceptable.

	Yes	No	Age or Date
1. Mumps	[ ]	[ ]	_____
2. Scarlet Fever	[ ]	[ ]	_____
3. Rheumatic Fever	[ ]	[ ]	_____
4. Hay Fever	[ ]	[ ]	_____
5. Asthma	[ ]	[ ]	_____
6. Bronchitis	[ ]	[ ]	_____
7. Pneumonia	[ ]	[ ]	_____
8. Pleurisy	[ ]	[ ]	_____
9. Tuberculosis	[ ]	[ ]	_____
10. Histoplasmosis	[ ]	[ ]	_____
11. Mononucleosis	[ ]	[ ]	_____
12. Sickle-Cell Disease	[ ]	[ ]	_____
13. Polio	[ ]	[ ]	_____
14. Meningitis	[ ]	[ ]	_____
15. Encephalitis	[ ]	[ ]	_____
16. High Blood Pressure	[ ]	[ ]	_____
17. Coronary Artery Disease	[ ]	[ ]	_____
18. Heart Attack	[ ]	[ ]	_____
19. Angina Pectoris	[ ]	[ ]	_____
20. Other Heart Disease	[ ]	[ ]	_____
21. Heart Murmer	[ ]	[ ]	_____

22. Arteriosclerosis [ ] [ ] _____

23. Stroke [ ] [ ] _____

24. Other Vascular Diseases [ ] [ ] _____

25. Thrombophlebitis [ ] [ ] _____

26. Emphysema [ ] [ ] _____

27. Other Lung Disease [ ] [ ] _____

28. Gallbladder Disease [ ] [ ] _____

29. Gallstones [ ] [ ] _____

30. Pancreatic Disease [ ] [ ] _____

31. Yellow Jaundice [ ] [ ] _____

32. Liver Disease [ ] [ ] _____

33. Chronic Gastritis [ ] [ ] _____

34. Gastric Ulcer [ ] [ ] _____

35. Appendicitis [ ] [ ] _____

36. Colitis [ ] [ ] _____

37. Duodenal Ulcer [ ] [ ] _____

38. Diverticulosis [ ] [ ] _____

39. Hernia [ ] [ ] _____

40. Diabetes [ ] [ ] _____

41. Hypoglycemia [ ] [ ] _____

42. Gout [ ] [ ] _____

43. Arthritis [ ] [ ] _____

44. Goiter [ ] [ ] _____

45. Thyroid Disorder [ ] [ ] _____

46. Bone Disease [ ] [ ] _____

47. Anemia [ ] [ ] _____

48. Polycythemia [ ] [ ] _____

49. Bleeding Disorder [ ] [ ] _____

50. Migraine [ ] [ ] _____

52. Epliepsy/Seizures [ ] [ ] _____

53. Fainting Spells	[ ]	[ ]	_____
54. Cancer	[ ]	[ ]	_____
55. Benign Tumors	[ ]	[ ]	_____
56. Glaucoma	[ ]	[ ]	_____
57. Other Eye Disease	[ ]	[ ]	_____

Other Medical Conditions

Have you had, or do you now have, any serious or major medical problems or illnesses (as differentiated from injuries and operations) that were not included anywhere above? If so, please list them below, followed by your age or the year when they occurred or first developed. If not, please write "none" in the space provided.

1. _____

2. _____

3. _____

4. _____

Operations

Have you undergone any of the operations listed below? If not, write "no" in the "Age or Date" column. If so, enter your age or the year when the operation was performed, and the name and location of the hospital. If you have had any other operations, please indicate the type in the list below.

Type of Operation	Age or Date	Hospital/Location
1. Tonsillectomy		
2. Appendectomy		
3. Hernia Repair		
4.		
5.		
6.		

Injuries or Accidents

Have you had any serious injuries or accidents? If so, list below, followed by your age or the year when they occurred. If not, write "none" below.

1. _____

2. _____

3. _____

4. _____

Drugs and Medications

What prescription or nonprescription medications are you presently taking (antihypertension, antihistamines, tranquilizers, pain medications, hormones, etc.):

_____

_____

_____

Allergies

Do you have any known allergies (e.g., penicillin, sulfa drugs, other antibiotics or drugs)? If so, please list them below. If not, write "none" below.

_____

_____

_____

Family History

If a brother, sister, mother, or father have had any of the following diseases, please note and state relationship.

1. Cancer _____

2. Tuberculosis _____

3. Diabetes _____

4. High Blood Pressure _____

5. Heart Disease _____

6. Kidney Stones _____

7. Kidney Disease _____

8. Other _____

Life-style

1. Please indicate the amount and quantity of consumption or use of the following:

a. Tobacco _____

b. Alcohol _____

c. Tranquilizers _____

d. Sleeping Pills _____

e. Coffee _____

f. Other _____

g. Other _____

2. If your current (or past) occupation has necessitated exposure to radiation, hazardous substances, or mechanical vibrations, please describe.

_____
_____
_____

3. Are you, or have you ever been, excessively overweight (obese)?

_____
_____
_____

4. Do you regularly exercise? Please describe.

_____
_____
_____

SUPPORT GROUPS AND INFORMATION SOURCES

The following is a list of organizations and individuals, as of late 1993, providing support, assistance, and general information to men with sexual dysfunction problems and their partners. In addition, many hospitals and medical groups, located in larger urban areas, now sponsor useful informational seminars on the subject that are typically free and open to all interested individuals. The health section of your local newspaper, particularly on weekends, may carry announcements of such events.

SELF-HELP SUPPORT GROUPS

Impotence Anonymous/Impotence Institute of America
Impotence Anonymous (I.A.), established in 1981, is a
self-help group for men with about 75 local chapters. Chapters are located in most major metropolitan centers. I-Anon
is a parallel organization for partners. Impotence Anonymous is affiliated with the Impotence Institute of America,
Inc., Washington, D.C., founded in 1983. The Institute is a
nonprofit organization dedicated to furthering the interests
of men with impotence problems and their families. The
organization also represents physicians specializing in male
sexual dysfunction and a number of private companies
manufacturing products for treating dysfunction.

To obtain the location of the nearest chapter of Impotence
Anonymous, referrals to appropriate physicians in your area
treating male sexual dysfunction, and free copies of useful Impotence Institute of America publications, write or telephone:

Impotence Institute of America, Inc.
2020 Pennsylvania Avenue, N.W., Suite 292
Washington, DC 20006
Telephone: (800) 669-1603

Information and assistance may also be obtained by
contacting the nearest Impotence Institute of America, Regional Medical Advisor, listed below:

Arizona–New Mexico

Michael A. Chasin, M.D.
Consultants in Urology, Ltd.
1500 South Dobson Road, Suite 315
Mesa, AZ 85202
Tel: (602) 834-0269

Arkansas

Steven K. Wilson, M.D.
2015 Chestnut
Van Buren, AR 72956
Tel: (501) 474-1225

Northern California

Robert S. Safran, M.D.
444 34th Street
Oakland, CA 94609
Tel: (510) 420-8114

Southern California–Southern Nevada

Stephen M. Auerbach, M.D.
400 Newport Center Drive, Suite 50
Newport Beach, CA 92662
Tel: (714) 644-7200

Florida

Richard L. Fein, M.D.
Fein & Winton Associates
12900 N.E. 17th Avenue, Suite 301
North Miami, FL 33181
Tel: (305) 891-5060

Georgia–Alabama

Steve Morganstern, M. D.
Morganstern Urology Clinic
3280 Howell Mill Road, Suite 125-West
Atlanta, GA 30327
Tel: (404) 352-8220
(800) 652-5644

Illinois–Indiana

Terry Mason, M.D.
Attention: Tom Bleser
8541 South State, Suite 9
Chicago, IL 60619
Tel: (312) 846-7000

Maryland–Delaware

Myron I. Murdock, M.D.
7500 Hanover Parkway, Suite 206
Greenbelt, MD 20770
Tel: (301) 441-8900

North Dakota–South Dakota–Montana–Wyoming–
Idaho

Manuel Neto, M.D.
P.O. Box 40
1500 24th Avenue, S.W.
Minot, ND 58702
Tel: (701) 852-6386

New Jersey

Matis A. Fermaglich, M.D.
865 Teaneck Road
Teaneck, NJ 07666-4513
Tel: (201) 837-0606

New York–Connecticut

Douglas Whitehead, M.D.
785 Park Avenue
New York, NY 10021
Tel: (212) 879-3131

Oklahoma–Kansas

James R. Leach, M.D.
1725 East 19th Street, Suite 801
Tulsa, OK 74104
Tel: (918) 749-8765

Pennsylvania

Alan N. Fleischer, M.D.
Urology Associates
200 North 13th Street, Suite 201
Reading, PA 19604
Tel: (215) 372-2351

Texas

David F. Mobley, M.D.
920 Frostwood, Suite 610
Houston, TX 77024
Tel: (713) 932-1819

Virginia–Washington, D.C.

David Schwartz, M.D.
5252 Dawes Avenue
Alexandria, VA 22311
Tel: (703) 998-7333

Not For Men Only

Not For Men Only, Chicago, Illinois, is a support group for men and their partners founded in 1984 by Dr. Terry Mason. The group has one chapter in Elmhurst, Illinois, which is also affiliated with Impotence Anonymous. Not For Men Only takes a multidisciplinary approach, which includes concern for psychological problems, and has a special orientation toward involvement of partners.

For information, write or telephone:

Not For Men Only
Mercy Hospital and Medical Center
Stevenson Expressway at King Drive
Chicago, IL 60616
Tel: (312) 567-5567

Potency Restored

Potency Restored, Silver Spring, Maryland, is a support group for couples established in 1981 by Dr. Guilio Scarzella, a Maryland urologist specializing in male sexual dysfunction. The group meets monthly and emphasizes a "total care" and "buddy system." Individual members are encouraged to develop ongoing relationships with other participants and to meet at other times than that of the regular monthly meeting to share mutual feelings and problems. Members of the group are encouraged to visit men while hospitalized for penile implants operations.

For information write or telephone:

Dr. Guilio Scarzella
Potency Restored
Montgomery Center, Suite 218
8630 Fenton Street
Silver Spring, MD 20910
Tel: (301) 588-5777

Recovery of Male Potency

Recovery of Male Potency (ROMP), Detroit, Michigan, is a support group established in 1983 by Cindy Meredith, R.N., a clinical nurse with a specialty in urology along with two men with a history of erectile dysfunction. ROMP activities are all conducted at medical facilities. Currently the organization numbers twenty-five self-help chapters throughout the United States.

For information, write or telephone:

Recovery of Male Potency (ROMP)
ROMP Center
Grace Hospital
18700 Meyers Road
Detroit, MI 48235
Tel: (800) TEL ROMP
(313) 927-3219 (in Michigan)

PROFESSIONAL ORGANIZATIONS

American Association of Sex Educators, Counselors
    and Therapists

The American Association of Sex Educators, Counselors and Therapists (AASECT), Chicago, Illinois, is a professional organization representing sex educators, counselors, therapists, and others with an interest in the study and treatment of sexual problems. The organization maintains a national register of individuals meeting professional standards for membership and can provide assistance in finding a sex therapist in your area.

For information, write or telephone:

American Association of Sex Educators, Counselors and
Therapists
435 North Michigan Ave., Suite 1717
Chicago, IL 60611
Tel: (312) 644-0828

American Urological Association

The American Urological Association (AUA), Baltimore, Maryland, founded in 1902, is the principal professional society in the urology field. More than 6,000 physicians specializing in various aspects of urology are members. The AUA has eight regional sections representing members in the United States, Canada, Mexico, Central America, and the Pacific and Caribbean regions.

For information (including address and phone numbers of the nearest AUA regional section), write or telephone:

American Urological Association
1120 North Charles Street
Baltimore, MD 21201
Tel: (410) 727-1100

COMPANY-SPONSORED INFORMATION SERVICES

Impotence Information Center, American Medical Systems
American Medical Systems, Minnetonka, Minnesota, a unit of the large pharmaceutical company, Pfizer, Inc., is a leading manufacturer of medical devices, including penile prostheses. The Impotence Information Center operated by the company offers valuable free information to the general public on impotence and assistance in contacting local support groups.

For information, write or telephone:

Impotence Information Center
American Medical Systems
Minneapolis, MN 55440
Telephone (800) 543-9632

Osborn Medical Systems
Osborn Medical Systems, Augusta, Georgia, is a manufacturer of external vacuum devices used to overcome erectile failure. The company offers a free information service in connection with all aspects of impotence and detailed data

about external vacuum therapy. Referrals to medical specialists in your area are also provided.

For information, write or telephone:

Osborn Medical Systems
P.O. Box 1478
Augusta, GA 30903
Tel: (800) 438-8592

Palisades Pharmaceutical

Palisades Pharmaceutical, Inc., Tenafly, New Jersey, is a manufacturer of a yohambine drug sold under the Yocon trade name. The company provides information on the drug and where treatment is available.

For information, write or telephone:

Palisades Pharmaceutical, Inc.
64 North Summit Street
Tenafly, NJ 07670
Tel: (800) 237-9083

DRUGS USED TO TREAT IMPOTENCE AND OTHER MALE SEXUAL DYSFUNCTION PROBLEMS

The following is a list of medications that have been cited in this book as being of potential value in the treatment of male sexual dysfunction. For each entry, we have shown the generic (chemical) name, the principal manufacturers' proprietary brand names, information on the most serious or relevant side effects, important precautions when using, and other relevant comments.

Generic Name	Brand Name(s)	Side Effects and Comments
Bromoscriptine mesylate	Parodel	Drug derived from ergot, used largely for treating Parkinson's disease and acromegaly. As the drug counters hyperprolactinemia, its use may also help to improve erectile function. Important side effects include nausea, headache, dizziness, and fatigue.
—	Ceritine	Name given to a mixture of papaverine and five other vasoactive agents used in penile injection therapy to improve erectile function. Only for use under a urolgist's supervision.
Fluoxetine hydrochloride	Prozac	A drug primarily that is used largely for treating depression. Also found to be effective in treating many cases of premature ejaculation. Should not be used simultaneously with any drug of the monamine oxidase inhibitor type. Side effects can include skin rashes, nervousness, and anxiety.
Levodopa	Larodopa, Sinemet	Drug used primarily for the treatment of Parkinson's disease. As the drug has been linked to priapism, it is being investigated as a possible medication for impotence. Side effects include involuntary movements, mental changes, convulsions, and nausea.

Minoxidil	Loniten, Rogaine	Vasoactive drug originally used for treatment of high blood pressure (Loniten). Now also used as topical treatment for baldness (Rogaine). Topical application of minoxidil to the penis has promise as an impotence treatment. Side effects of topical application of Rogaine include skin irritation and rashes, respiratory and gastrointestinal problems, headache, and dizziness.
Naloxon	Narcan	Drug primarily used for the treatment of opiod narcotic depression. Use may improve erectile function. Side effects include nausea, sweating, tremulousness, and cardiovascular symptoms.
Nitroglycerine	—	Drug usually used mainly in patch form for relief from the pain of angina pectoris. Under investigation as a treatment for impotence. Side effects include headaches and dizziness.
Oxytocin	Pitocin, Syntocinon	Drug used to induce labor in pregnant women. May help to improve erectile function. Side effects include cardiac arrhythmia and nausea.
Papaverine	Cerebid	Penile injection drug. Should be used only under a urologist's supervision, due to possibility of episodes of priapism or penile scarring. The drug is available under other brand names. Sometimes used in combinations with other drugs.

Pentoxifylline	Trental	Drug primarily used for the treatment of arterial disease. Has been found in some cases to improve erectile function. Side effects can include gastrointestinal problems, dizziness, headache, tremor, and chest pain.
Phentolamine	Regitine	Penile injection drug. Should be used only under a urologist's supervision, due to possibility of episodes of priapism or penile scarring. Sometimes used in combination with other drugs.
Potassium p-aminobenzoate	Potaba	Drug used to treat Peyronie's disease. Side effects may include anorexia, nausea, fever, and rash. Should not be used when taking any sulfonamide drug.
Propylthiouracil	Propylthiouracil	Drug that counters the effects of hyperthyroidism, including loss of libido and erectile problems. Most serious side effect is agranulocytosis, the destruction of white blood cells with resulting impairment of the immune system. When taking, always promptly report any symptoms of illness to your physician.
Prostaglandin E_1	Alprostadil	Penile injection drug. Should be used only under urologist's supervision, due to possibility of episodes of priapism or penile scarring. Sometimes used in combination with other drugs.

Trazodone	Desyrel	Drug used in higher dosages as an antidepressant. In lower dosages, will sometime help to improve erectile function. May cause episodes of cardiac arrhythmia. Trazodone is sometimes used in combination with yohimbine. Do not drink alcohol when taking drug.
Testosterone cypionate	Depo-Testosterone /Virilon IM	For intramuscular injection. Should be used only under a physician's direction. Not for use in any patient with evidence of a prostate tumor.
Testosterone enanthate	Delatestryl	For intramuscular injection. Should be used only under a physician's direction. Not for use in any patient with evidence of a prostate tumor.
Vasoactive intestinal polypeptide	—	A hormone used in combination with phentoalamine in penile injection therapy. Also known as VIP.
Yohimbine hydrochloride	Yocon/Yohimex/ Dayto Himbin/ Aphrodyne	Drug with apparent aphrodisiac properties. May cause elevated blood pressure, rapid heart rate, irritability, tremor, dizziness, headache, and nausea.

Tips for a Sexually Healthy Diet

In general, the best diet from the standpoint of preventing erectile dysfunction is one that will also protect the health of your cardiovascular system. This follows from the fact that defects in the cardiovascular system are among the principal causes of impotence and, fortunately, a class of disorder where prevention can pay off.

A diet that will help to prevent both cardiovascular problems and male sexual dysfunction will have the following goals:

◆ Provide only enough daily calories to maintain proper body weight in relation to your height and build (generally within the 2,000- to 2,500-calorie range)

- Contain an optimum balance of protein, carbohydrates, and fats
- Provide a minimum quantity of cholesterol
- Supply most fats in the polyunsaturated form
- Provide adequate vitamins, particularly vitamins A (ideally in beta carotene form), C, and E
- Provide an adequate supply of minerals
- Contain adequate fiber
- Provide meals that are interesting, varied, and tasty

This appendix provides lists of foods that will help you achieve the dietary goals indicated. It also contains lists of foods to avoid, or at least to limit, and some tips on special problems such as eating out. It is worth noting that a proper diet, suitably prepared, also can be very tasty.

SOME SEXUALLY HEALTHY FOODS

High-Protein Group

Chicken—preferably not fried and always with the skin removed

Turkey

Fish—all types, preferably steamed or broiled

Shellfish—steamed or broiled in moderate quantities

Red meats—no more than 7 ounces per day of veal, beef, pork, lamb, or game (only use when well trimmed and lean)

Tofu—excellent when lightly stir fried with vegetables

Dried peas and beans

Peanut butter—avoid if you have a peanut butter allergy

High-Carbohydrate Group

Hot and cold breakfast cereals—preferably high-fiber types with no sugar added

Breakfast grits

Whole wheat, rye, pumpernickel, and other dark breads

Whole wheat rolls, English muffins, and bagels

Low-fat, minimum-sugar baked goods—try angel food cake, pretzels, rice cake, and soda and graham crackers

Popcorn—avoid added butter or oil

Pasta—all types

Fats and Oils Group

Unsalted margarine—only in moderate quantity as a spread; look for brands made from sunflower, safflower, canola, and corn oil.

Cooking oils high in monounsaturated fats—olive and peanut oil (Note: Always use liquid oils for cooking in preference to butter, margarine, or shortenings.)

Cooking oils high in polyunsaturated fats—corn, soybean, sunflower, and safflower oils

Salad oils high in monounsaturated fats—see above

Salad oils high in polyunsaturated fats—see above.

Dairy Product Group

Skimmed or 1 percent low-fat liquid milk

Powdered nonfat or low-fat milk

Cheese—low-fat cottage, mozzarella, ricotta, Swiss, and other white-colored varieties

Yogurt—low-fat varieties

Ice milk, sherbet, and sorbet

Fruit and Vegetable Group

Raw fruits—all types, especially good when served in mixed salad form and without addition of dairy toppings or sugar (try adding a very small amount of an appropriate cordial)

Cooked and canned fruits—preferably unsweetened

Raw vegetables—all types, especially good when served in mixed salad form with small amounts of olive oil and vinegar

Cooked and canned vegetables—all types, but especially cabbage, brussels sprouts, broccoli, and cauliflower (add only small quantities of suitable fats and oils)

Vegetable soups

Rice and potatoes—add only small quantities of suitable fats and oils

Fruit and vegetable juices, preferably unsweetened

SOME FOODS TO EAT IN LIMITED QUANTITY OR ON SPECIAL OCCASIONS

High-Protein Group

Fatty red meats—bacon, sausage, marbled beef, high-fat hamburger, and most processed cold cuts

Pickled meats—corned beef and pastrami

Fried chicken, fish, and shellfish (especially breaded)

Duck and goose

Egg yolks (no limit on white portion of eggs)

Liver and most variety meats

High-Carbohydrate Group

High-fat pasta and rice products

High-fat snack foods—pork rinds, potato chips, cheese crackers

High-fat cakes, cookies, pastry, and doughnuts

Fats and Oils Group

Margarine—all products made largely from hydrogenated oils or partially hydrogenated vegetable oils or animal fats

Shortenings—all products made largely from hydrogenated or partially hydrogenated vegetable oils or animal fats

Chocolate

Sour cream or cheese-type salad dressings

Dairy Products Group

Butter

High-fat milk, cream, including whipped and sour cream

High-fat ice cream

High-fat cheese—including many yellow cheeses

High-fat yogurt

Fruit and Vegetable Group

Avocado (due to high fat content)

Vegetables—all cooked or seasoned with butter, lard, hydrogenated shortening, deep fat, chunks of pork fat, and cream sauces

Vegetables marinated in oil

Beverages Group

Alcohol (Alcoholism is an important factor in impotence. Alcohol can also cause prostate irritation.)

Coffee, tea, and soft drinks containing caffeine (can irritate the prostate. Note: Very spicy foods can also cause prostate irritation.)

SOME FOODS TO BE AVOIDED OR KEPT TO THE ABSOLUTE MINIMUM

Cocoa butter

Shredded coconut (in any form)—coconut cakes, cookies, and candy

Coconut oil

Palm and palm kernel oils

Margarine and shortenings made from coconut, palm, and palm kernel oils

Heavy cream

TIPS WHEN EATING OUT

Tip 1: Don't hesitate to ask questions or ask for your food to be prepared the proper way when eating out.

Comment: Eating out presents a real problem in trying to maintain a sexually healthy diet. Not only is there a tendency to eat too much, in terms of total calories, but typical restaurant food is often high in cholesterol and saturated fats. There is very little that you can do when your choice is limited to eating fast food or going hungry. At any better restaurant, you should not hesitate to ask how any menu item is normally prepared and, when indicated, request that it be prepared in a healthier manner. Also, always request that any sauces be served separately so that you can control the amount added to your food.

Tip 2: Be especially careful about breakfast.

Comment: Of all the meals you eat out, breakfast usually presents the most difficulty. Largely for economic reasons, the typical American restaurant usually limits your choice of breakfast entree to fried eggs; pancakes, waffles, and other items containing eggs; and bacon and sausage. Any accompanying toast is usually served soaked in butter. Ask whether there is any cold or hot cereal available or some fresh fruit. If everything else fails, buy some juice, fruit, and bran muffins at the nearest convenience store and eat in your room or car.

Tip 3: Look for seafood and vegetarian restaurants.

Comment: Seafood and vegetarian food can be a good choice when eating out, both from the standpoint of taste and health. At seafood restaurants, however, insist that your entree be broiled, baked, or steamed. Heavily breaded and deep-fried seafood is a serious mistake. At vegetarian restaurants, be sure to check whether any item is prepared with sour cream or cheese.

Tip 4: Look for certain ethnic restaurants.

Comment: Most authentic Asian food, whether Chinese, Japanese, Indian, Thai, or Vietnamese, is largely a mixture of vegetables over a bed of rice or noodles. Relatively small amounts of meat are typically added, with the meat principally serving to provide flavor. When ordering Asian cuisine, be sure that no coconut oil is used in the preparation, and avoid items that have a high oil content in general. Italian food is a good choice as most of any meals usually feature pasta and olive oil is used in cooking. Mexican food is largely based on dried beans and corn with meat portions at a minimum. Limit your consumption of guacamole, as it contains avocado, and Mexican items with sour cream.

Tip 5: Try to avoid buffets and salad bars.

Comment: The problem with salad bars and buffets is that there is a tendency always to eat too much. Many of the food choices are high in fat and cholesterol. If you have no choice but to eat at a buffet or salad bar, check out the entire selection of foods first and then select only the healthier items in moderation.

Tip 6: Check your airline before flying to see if any special meals are available.

Comment: Most travelers don't realize that many airlines serve special meals, including meals of a vegetarian, fresh fruit, low-calorie, and seafood nature. Such meals usually have to be ordered in advance. A plus is that these special meals are often much better than the usual airline fare.

Tip 7: Just try to do your best when it comes to special events.

Comment: Special events, such as family and social gatherings, major annual holidays, office parties, and other business functions all present an almost unsurmountable challenge to maintaining a diet conducive to your sexual health. Unless you must attend such events on a very frequent basis, just do the best you can and go back to your healthy diet the very next day. If such events are frequent and unavoidable, a special effort of will power is required.

Finally, there are the endless challenges presented by annual holidays, such as Thanksgiving and Christmas, special family occasions, office parties, and social events. There is no easy solution to these problems. The best advice is to accept the inevitability of these occasions, but afterward promptly resume your healthy diet. Continuing to maintain your exercise program, as discussed in other chapters, also will help.

EXERCISE AND MALE SEXUAL HEALTH

This appendix discusses two types of exercises that will benefit male sexual performance. The first are exercises designed to improve your overall cardiovascular fitness. Such exercises serve to prevent the deterioration of the vascular system serving your penis, which, of course, is a critical element in proper erectile function. They are also an important factor in weight control. The second are exercises designed to enhance the flexibility and tone of the muscles of the lower abdominal area and vicinity of the penis. Such exercises help to maintain a healthy form of blood flow in the genital region.

Cardiovascular Fitness Exercise Programs

Exercises that improve cardiovascular fitness are those that safely and comfortably increase heart rate and breathing for a period of time of at least 20 minutes. Such exercises help to prevent erectile dysfunction as they lessen the possibility of plaque formation in the arteries supplying blood to the penis and maintain blood vessel flexibility. If you have led a fairly sedentary existence in the past, the most appropriate types of exercises to consider when deciding on doing something about your cardiovascular fitness are, in order of desirability, swimming, walking, and aerobics.

The following are some relevant observations regarding each:

Swimming. Swimming involves virtually no pain and very little danger of injury to the skeletal system, muscles, and joints. It is also pleasurable and a good way to relieve tensions. A 30-minute swim daily is ideal. Cardiovascular benefits are obtainable from as few as three 30-minute swims each week. Each swim should be conducted on a leisurely, but continuously moving, basis, and there is little reason to engage in very vigorous "lap" swimming.

Walking. While not everybody has access to a swimming pool, there is always a place to walk. Walking at least 2 miles each day at a brisk pace, with only brief and occasional pauses for rest, is recommended. With proper conditioning, long hikes of up to 10 miles a day are both beneficial and enjoyable. Walking presents little chance of injury just as long as you remember to wear proper shoes and avoid walking during times of the day when heat and humidity are excessive.

Aerobics. Aerobics are series of exercises designed to systematically raise your heart and breathing rates for an extended period of time. Aerobics may be performed on your own, but they are most effective, and usually the most enjoyable, when performed in a class setting with a qualified instructor. In the classroom setting, aerobics are typically performed to music. Each session, which generally lasts about an hour, starts with a warm-up phase designed to heat and stretch important muscle groups. The warm-up is followed by an approximately 20-minute period of active exercise intended to raise your heart rate to a level suitable for your age group. The session concludes with a series of exercises designed to tone certain muscles such as the abdominals. Three aerobic sessions per week of the low-impact type should yield cardiovascular benefits.

Flexibility and Toning Exercises

Exercises designed to enhance the tone and flexibility of blood vessels and muscles in the genital area contain elements of muscular stretching, contraction, and relaxation. With the exception of Kegel exercises, which are discussed shortly, many of these elements are often incorporated into the standard one-hour aerobic class session.

In stretching exercises, individual muscle groups are subjected to a brief period of tension followed by a period of relaxation. This, in time, will loosen the tendons and muscles that control the range of motion around some individual joint in the body and allow for a full range of motion of that joint. Stretching can be of several types. Dynamic stretches are exercises characterized by smooth, gentle movements of some part of the body. Tightening and relaxation stretching is characterized by cycles of up to 30 seconds of muscular tension followed by 2- or 3-second periods of relaxation. Bounce stretching, also known as ballistic stretching, consists of a series of pulselike stretches, with part of the body being exercised at its point of maximum normal range. Most authorities recommend caution while performing bounce stretching exercises.

The following are some specific exercises that can easily be performed at home and that should serve to improve the tone and flexibility of the muscles and blood vessels in your genital region:

Abdominal Control Exercises. Abdominal control exercises are designed to control the abdominal muscles. Appropriate exercises exist for the entire range of abdominal muscles; however, the most relevant, from the standpoint of male sexual function, are those designed to strengthen the lower abdominal muscles in the vicinity of the groin. Strengthening the lower abdominal muscles serves to keep the internal organs of the pelvic area in place. They also help to strengthen the lower back.

To exercise the lower abdominal muscles, lie flat on your back with your feet on the floor and your knees raised and positioned apart. Then tighten and relax your lower abdominal muscles. When you are performing the exercise correctly, you should experience a slight upward movement of your hips and feel the small of your back push against the floor each time you tense the muscles. The exercise should be repeated at least ten times per exercise cycle. Only a small move is required each time you tighten the abdominal muscles.

Another simple exercise for the lower abdominal muscles can be performed in a standing position. Stand erect, feet slightly apart, and with knees slightly bent. Then place your hands together behind your head as if holding a sledge hammer. Then quickly move your hands forward and suddenly stop when your hands are immediately above your head. The result should be a quick contraction of the muscles of your lower abdomen. The exercise should be repeated about ten times.

Cat Stretches. Cat stretches are performed on your hands and knees and facing down on the floor. While in this position, arch and stretch your back upward, while simultaneously exhaling. Then, while inhaling, return slowly to the original position. Repeat the exercise about ten times. When performed correctly, cat stretches will help to strengthen the overall pelvic area, as well as prove beneficial to the back.

Kegal Exercises. Kegel exercises were originally developed by Dr. Arnold H. Kegel, a gynecologist, as a means for controlling incontinence in women. There have been reports that men who practice Kegel exercises can improve male sexual function.

Kegel exercises consist of a series of tightening and relaxation of the pubococcygeus muscle. This muscle, located in the vicinity of the rectum, is the muscle that you can feel tensing whenever you attempt to start the flow of urine, while voiding, or attempt to shut off the flow. The simplest way to perform a Kegel exercise is while seated in a cross-legged position. While in this position, pull upward on your anal region as if attempting to contain a bowel movement. Hold this position for about ten seconds and then relax. Each Kegel exercise cycle should consist of at least ten upward pulls, with corresponding periods of relaxation.

Pelvic Thrusts. A pelvic thrust is a simple exercise that helps to improve the tone of the muscles in the lower pelvic area. The exercise can be easily performed while in a seated position, by simultaneously squeezing the buttocks together, pulling inward on the area of the anus and the lower abdomen, and thrusting the entire pelvic area forward. The overall motions are similar to the movements made by a male during sexual intercourse.

To perform pelvic thrusts properly, each thrust should be held for a period of several seconds. Each thrust should then be followed by a brief period of relaxation. An ideal exercise cycle would consist of about ten complete thrusts. An excellent time to perform pelvic thrusts is when seated for long periods while traveling. In such circumstances, pelvic thrusts can help to overcome some of the stiffness associated with extended travel. Another good time to practice pelvic thrusts is while swimming.

Pelvic lifts are a related exercise that provides some benefit to the pelvic area. To perform a pelvic lift, first lie flat on your back, legs parallel, knees bent upward and arms outstretched. Then lift your pelvic area upward, while supporting yourself on your feet and back. While raising upward, the body should be kept in a straight line from the shoulder area to the knees.

Squats. Squats are exercises designed to improve the general muscle tone of the lower pelvic area. In performing a single sitting squat, lower yourself slowly into a sitting position with your buttocks pointed downward and your knees pointed upward. While doing this, it is essential that both your feet, including your heels, rest flat on the floor. While squatting, it is all right to rest your arms or hands lightly on your knees in order to maintain balance. You should perform about ten squats during each exercise cycle.

Yoga. Yoga is a series of physical exercises, with philosophical overtones, developed in India. Yoga combines meditations with various traditional physical postures and controlled breathing. Individuals who regularly practice yoga often gain excellent suppleness and flexibility, including in the pelvic region. As yoga takes a fair amount of commitment, it will probably not be worth the time as a means for maintaining male sexual function, unless you happen to enjoy the overall experience.

GLOSSARY OF MALE SEXUAL DYSFUNCTION TERMS

A

Adrenal glands: A pair of small ductless glands located on the top of each kidney. Hormones secreted by the adrenal glands include epinephrine (adrenalin), norepinephrine (noradrenalin), hydrocortisone, and the sex hormones testosterone and estrogen.

Adrenaline: *See* Epinephrine

Androgen hormone: A type of hormone produced in the body that plays an essential role in the normal development and performance of the male sexual organs; also essential to the development of normal secondary male sexual characteristics, including facial and body hair, muscular structure, and deep voice. Testosterone, produced in the testicles and the adrenal glands, is the most important androgen hormone.

Antiandrogen drug: A drug that is prescribed to totally block or significantly reduce the normal activity of an androgen hormone. The side effects of such drugs, which are often used in the treatment of prostate gland tumors (both benign and malignant prostate), may include loss of libido (sexual desire) and erectile dysfunction.

Antihistamine: A drug mainly used to counter the effects of high levels of histamine in the body. A histamine buildup occurs in the body when an allergic reaction results after exposure to pollen and other substances. In some men, the taking of prescription or over-the-counter antihistamines may result in erectile dysfunction.

Anti-inflammatory drug: Any drug taken to counter pain, swelling, heat, and other irritation due to infection or another cause.

Arteriography: A radiological diagnostic procedure used to determine the condition of the interior of an artery. The procedure is invasive in nature as it requires the injection of a substance into the bloodstream that enhances X-ray images. An arteriogram is sometimes ordered when there is reason to believe that impotence is due to a blockage in an artery supplying the penis.

Artery: A blood vessel that carries blood under pressure away from the heart to all parts of the body. A restriction in the flow of blood in the arteries supplying the penis can result in erectile dysfunction.

Atherosclerosis: A cardiovascular disease in which cholesterol and other fatty deposits accumulate within arteries and impair blood flow. The condition is often referred to as hardening of the arteries.

Autonomic nervous system: That portion of the body's peripheral nervous system that controls activities that are generally beyond conscious control, including respiration, the pumping action of the heart, and the process of erection.

B

Behavior therapy: A treatment procedure employing behavioral psychology principles in which patients are systematically subjected to conditioning of a stimulus and response nature to obtain relief from a problem with no known physical cause. Has been used with mixed results in treating psychological impotence.

Benign prostatic hyperplasia (BPH): Also known as benign prostate hypertropy, a condition characterized by the growth of a benign (noncancerous) tumor inside the prostate gland. The treatment of the condition by surgery or drugs can sometimes result in erectile dysfunction

Beta carotene: A nontoxic form of vitamin A found naturally in many fruits and vegetables; also the coloring agent added to margarine to obtain a yellow color. There is increasing evidence that taking beta carotene, due to its antioxidant properties, can help slow down the aging process.

Biofeedback: A treatment method involving training patients to control some area of bodily activity such as temperature or blood pressure by observing and reacting to sight or sound signals. The technique has been used in the treatment of erectile problems with mixed results.

Biothesiometry: A noninvasive test in which a special device is employed that subjects the skin of the penis to a controlled series of vibrations. The degree of sensitivity of the penis skin to vibrations is an indication of the health of the sensory nerves of the organ.

Bladder: Stretchable, pouchlike organ located inside the pelvic cavities of both men and women that temporarily stores of urine produced in the kidneys.

Blood count: A type of blood test performed to determine the level of red and white blood cells and platelets in the blood stream. An abnormal blood count may indicate that the patient has an infection or some form of anemia. Bloods count are routinely run when investigating an impotence problem.

Blood poisoning: An infection that occurs when the bloodstream is invaded by bacteria or fungi. The condition, also known as septicemia, may follow surgical treatments for impotence, but is usually easily treated.

Blood test: Any test performed on a sample of a patient's blood. When treating impotence, the series of blood tests performed may include a blood count; sedimentation rate measurement; and the determination of blood levels of sugar, cholesterol, and triglycerides. When an infection is suspected, the blood may be tested to determine the identity of any pathogenic organism present.

Bulbocavernosus (BC) reflex test: A test that can be performed at home to determine whether there is normal nerve function in the penis and vicinity. The test involves the quick squeezing of the tip of the penis and observing whether a simultaneous contraction is felt in the anus.

Bulbous urethra: An enlarged section of the urethra (urinary passage) where seminal fluid temporarily collects while the penis is stimulated prior to ejaculation. The bulbous urethra is located below the point where the urethra passes through the prostate gland.

Bypass surgery: Surgery performed to provide a pathway for blood flow around a blockage in an artery. Bypass surgery is sometimes used to treat blood flow problems in the arteries supplying the penis.

C

Cancer: A disease in which there is the uncontrolled growth of abnormal cell tissue in some part of the body along with the possibility that the condition will spread from its initial site of origin to other parts of the body and prove life threatening. Prostate cancer is a very common condition in older men. Impotence can be a side effect of the surgical, radiological, and hormonal treatment of prostate cancer.

Cardiovascular disease: Any disease that impairs the functioning of the heart and the blood circulatory system. Erectile dysfunction can be a consequence of a cardiovascular disease affecting the flow of blood into and away from the penis.

Castration: The surgical removal of the testicles (also known as orchiectomy) to eliminate the main source of testosterone. Castration is sometimes employed in the treatment of prostate cancer. The use of certain antiandrogen drugs that block testosterone is now sometimes referred to as chemical castration.

Cavernosal artery: The main artery through which blood flows into the erectile tissues of the penis.

Cavernosography: An invasive radiological procedure used to determine the site or sites of blood leakage from the penis during erection. The procedure, which is usually performed with the penis in an erect state, requires the injection of an imaging substance.

Central nervous system: That portion of the nervous system consisting of the brain and the nerve fibers of the spinal cord.

Chlamydia: An infectious disease that most often appears as a vaginal infection in women. Men can be infected, with a whitish penile discharge a typical symptom. The sexual transmission of the disease can result in a form of prostatitis in men, along with premature ejaculation problems.

Cholesterol: A steroid chemical substance produced naturally by the body or obtained by eating certain foods. Cholesterol, in excess of that normally needed by the body, can cause a variety of health problems, including cardiovascular disease, often a factor in impotence.

Circumcision: In men, the surgical removal of the foreskin (part of the forward tip of the penis). Circumcision originally evolved as a religious practice, but it is now routinely performed on most American males. Circumcision may be recommended in men where an unusually tight foreskin prevents erection or causes discomfort during erection.

Coitus interruptus: The deliberate removal of the penis from a woman's vagina prior to ejaculation. The practice is not recommended for birth control, due to its high failure rate. Coitus interruptus may also result in a prostate congested with seminal fluid and associated pain and irritation.

Coliform bacteria: Bacteria normally present in the gastrointestinal systems of humans and other animals. When coliform bacteria invades the prostate, the result can be the most common type of prostate infection and a cause of premature ejaculation.

Congestion: The buildup of fluid in some part of the body. When congestion occurs in the prostate, the result can be pain and irritation. Certain sexual practices can cause prostate congestion.

Corpus cavernosagram: *See* Cavernosography

Corpus cavernosum: Two parallel pairs of erectile tissues inside the penis containing thousands of expandable saclike cavities (sinuses). An erection takes place when blood fills and is retained in the cavities.

Corpus spongiosum: The cylindrically shaped structure in the penis surrounding the urethra and extending over the length of the penis.

D

Deep dorsal vein: The large vein that carries blood away from the penis. Blood flows in the deep dorsal vein from the large number of smaller veins inside the erectile tissues

Diabetes mellitus: A very common disease characterized by the inability of the pancreas to produce a sufficient quantity of the hormone insulin for the digestion of glucose, a sugar providing most of the energy required by the body. Diabetes is a major cause of impotence.

Diagnosis: A medical explanation and conclusion of the cause of some form of medical disorder, based upon the observation of signs and symptoms and, where indicated, scientific tests.

Digital rectal examination: An examination conducted to determine the health of the prostate, including the presence of a benign or malignant prostate tumor or a prostate infection. In cases of premature ejaculation, the examination may include massage of the gland to obtain a sample of prostatic fluid for laboratory analysis to check for the presence of infectious organisms.

Diuretic: Any drug, food, or beverage that promotes the excretion of urine. Some diuretic drugs have been linked to erectile failure.

Dorsal artery: The main artery supplying blood to the penis. A blockage in the dorsal artery, due to plaque formation, may be the cause of erectile failure.

E

Ejaculate: The fluid that (except in the case of the condition know as retrograde ejaculation) normally is discharged by the penis during ejaculation. The ejaculate normally contains fluid produced in the testicles, seminal vesicles, and prostate gland.

Ejaculation: The discharge of seminal fluid from the penis due to sexual intercourse or masturbation. Ejaculation is caused by the contraction of muscles of the urethra and in the vicinity of the prostate.

Ejaculatory failure: The failure of a man to ejaculate and achieve orgasm, despite an extended period of erotic and physical stimulus of the penis.

Electrostimulation: A medical technique used to cause ejaculation based on the application of a mild electrical current to the nerve centers controlling the ejaculatory process.

Epididymis: One of two oblong structures attached to the back of each testicle that composes the first portion of the duct system that transports fluid produced in each testicle.

Epilepsy: A disease, usually associated with seizures, caused by some abnormality in the transmission of electrical signals between the nerve cells of the brain. Some drugs used to control epilepsy have been linked to erectile failure.

Epinephrine: A chemical substance, commonly known as adrenaline, that is produced by the adrenal glands. Epinephrine and norepinephrine (also produced by the adrenal glands) are important factors in the control of heart rate and blood pressure. Loss of erection can occur from a surge of epinephrine and norepinephrine due to the contraction of the smooth muscle tissue of the penis.

Erectile dysfunction: Another name for impotence. A panel of the National Institutes of Health has recommended the use of the term "erectile failure" in preference to impotence, due to the negative connotations of the latter.

Erection: The physical state of the penis resulting from the temporary absorption of blood inside the erectile tissues and characterized by increased penile length and rigidity.

Estrogen: A sex hormone that plays an important role in the development of female sexual characteristics. The ovaries of young women normally produce estrogen in large quantity. Smaller amounts are produced by the testicles of men. Estrogen therapy is sometimes prescribed in the treatment of prostate tumors and can cause erectile dysfunction and loss of libido as a side effect.

External device: A mechanical apparatus containing a pump that is designed to create a vacuum around the flaccid penis. The vacuum, in turn, serves to draw blood into the penis and results in an erection that can be temporarily sustained by a ring placed around the base of the penis.

F

Flaccid: The nonerect state of the penis characterized by an absence of sufficient rigidity to obtain penetration of the vagina.

Foreplay: Physical erotic stimulation preceding sexual intercourse. Extended foreplay not followed by ejaculation should be avoided as prostate congestion and irritation may be the result.

G

Glans: The medical name for the forwardmost portion or head of the penis.

Gonorrhea: A sexually transmitted disease, often referred to as "the clap." Gonorrhea may cause a form of prostatitis and result in premature and painful ejaculation. Any yellowish discharge from the penis should be promptly investigated and treated.

Groin: The portion of the lower abdomen located above the penis and where the thighs connect to the body. Stretching exercises that improve the tone of muscles and the organs in the groin area may play a positive role in the proper functioning of the urinary-genital system.

H

Herb: A natural product, obtained from a nonwoody plant, valued for its flavor, fragrance, or medicinal properties.

Herbal medicine: Medicine based on the use of natural herbal substances. Much of prescientific medicine was based on the use of herbs found by trial or error by folk practitioners to have desirable medical properties. Modern medicine, however, requires the systematic demonstration of medical properties under controlled clinical conditions.

High blood pressure: A disorder, medically known as hypertension and characterized by an excessive level of pressure within the blood circulatory system. Certain drugs used to treat high blood pressure have been linked to erectile failure.

Hormones: Chemical substances, essential to various biological processes, that are produced by different endocrine glands in the body.

Hormonal therapy: Medical treatment involving the administration of certain hormones or hormonal blocking drugs. Treatment of prostate tumors and other conditions with hormonal therapy may result in erectile dysfunction or loss of libido.

Hypertension: *See* High Blood Pressure

I

Infertility: In a male, some defect of the sperm or seminal fluid that results in inability to successfully impregnate a female partner. Not to be confused with impotence. Infertility may be desired as in the case of a man choosing a vasectomy.

Implant: A prothesis or artificial device that when surgically inserted into the penis will provide sufficient rigidity for vaginal penetration.

Impotence: The inability of a man to achieve or maintain an erection of sufficient duration for the satisfaction of both sexual partners.

Irritated prostate: A prostate problem characterized by pain and discomfort that is often the result of a man's pattern of sexual behavior.

K

Kegel exercises: Exercises of the pelvic area originally developed as a means for controlling urinary incontinence in women. The Kegel exercise system may also help to improve male sexual performance.

Kidneys: Two glandular organs that serve to separate waste products from the blood which are then eliminated from the body in the urine. The kidneys are located close to the spinal column and at the back of the abdominal cavity.

L

Lack of desire: Also known as loss of libido. A condition, often with a physical cause, characterized by the loss of sexual interest.

Libido: *See* Lack of desire.

Luteinizing hormone (LH): A type of hormone that serves to promote the secretion of male and female sex hormones. LH hormones are produced in the pituitary gland.

Luteinizing hormone-releasing hormone (LHRH) therapy: A type of hormone therapy that employs drugs known as LHRH analogs to block the action of testosterone and other sex hormones. When LHRH therapy is used in the treatment of prostate cancer, erectile dysfunction and loss of desire may be side effects.

M

Male sexual dysfunction: Any disorder of the male genital system that interferes with sexual performance, such as impotence and premature ejaculation.

Masturbation: Self-stimulation of sexual organs. In the male, masturbation is usually, but not always, accompanied by erection and ejaculation.

Minerals: Simple chemical substances that are essential in the diet of animals, including humans. About 30 essential minerals have been identified, some metallic compounds (calcium, iron, sodium, potassium, magnesium, copper, manganese, and zinc) and other nonmetallic (phosphorus, iodine, sulfur, chlorine, and fluorine).

Multiple sclerosis (MS): A disease of the nervous system usually characterized by progressive muscular weakness and loss of function. In men, impotence often results from the disease.

N

Nocturnal erections: Erections that occur normally and spontaneously while asleep, possibly accompanied by ejaculation.

Nocturnal penile tumescence (NPT) test: A test procedure that measures the presence, frequency, and physical characteristics of nocturnal erections. The test is noninvasive and is typically conducted in a sleep laboratory setting.

Nonprescription drug: A legally available drug that is sold without medical prescription. Also known as an over-the-counter drug.

O

Obesity: Excessive and unhealthy body weight. The National Institutes of Health defines obesity as weight equal to or in excess of 20 percent of an individual's body mass index (BMI). The BMI is the ratio of an individual's weight and height in kilograms per meter, as compared to a normal value in men of 24.

Orchiectomy: *See* Castration

Orgasm: In men, the pleasurable sensations usually felt in the penis during ejaculation. The sensations are associated with the vigorous contractions of muscles in the vicinity of the urethra and pelvic area. Orgasm is possible in men subject to erectile dysfunction. In the case of men subject to the condition known as retrograde ejaculation, orgasm can occur without the expulsion of ejaculate from the penis.

Outpatient: Treatment that takes place in a hospital or at a medical office and does not involve an overnight hospital stay.

P

Painful ejaculation: Ejaculation accompanied by pain and discomfort that are often caused by an infection of the prostate or seminal vesicles.

Papaverine: A smooth muscle relaxant drug that results in erection when injected into the penis. Papaverine is used in the diagnosis of erectile failure and in penile injection therapy.

Parasympathetic nervous system: That portion of the autonomic nervous system that is involved in the unconscious processes associated with erection.

Parkinson's disease: A disease characterized by the progressive degeneration of nerve centers within the brain. Erectile dysfunction has been linked to some of the drugs used for treatment of the disease.

Pelvic injuries: Physical injuries to the pelvic area resulting from accidents or surgical trauma. When pelvic injuries result in damage to the nerves or vascular system serving the penis, impotence may be a consequence.

Pelvic relaxation exercises: Exercises designed to improve the muscular tone of the pelvic region of the body; may have a positive effect on male sexual performance.

Pelvic thrusts: Physical movements involving the repeated forward thrusting of the pelvic region. Pelvic thrust exercises may have a positive effect on male sexual performance.

Pelvis: That skeletal area of the body where the lower or hind limbs join the trunk of the body and is in the form of a bony girdle.

Penile-brachial index: A measurement that compares the magnitude of the blood pressure in the penis with the blood pressure reading taken at about the same time from the arm and which serves as a possible indication of insufficient blood supply to the penis.

Penile implant: An artificial device or prothesis that when surgically inserted into the penis provides sufficient rigidity for vaginal penetration. Penile implants may be of the semirigid malleable, simple self-contained, or three-piece inflatable type.

Penile injection therapy: An impotence treatment in which a smooth muscle relaxant drug is injected into the penis to cause an erection of sufficient rigidity and duration for vaginal penetration and sexual intercourse.

Penile warts: Growths on the penis caused by a virus;. medically known as condylomas. The condition is normally harmless in men, but it should be treated due to an association with cervical cancer in female partners.

Penis: The organ in male animals used for the passage of urine and vaginal penetration during intercourse. The penis has both an external portion and a portion located inside the body.

Performance anxiety: An emotional condition in a man characterized by a reluctance to engage in sexual intercourse due to fear of failure and possible negative reaction of the female partner.

Perineal injury: An injury to the area of the body known as the perineum and which may result in sexual dysfunction.

Perineum: That portion of the lower end of the trunk of the body located between the rectum and the genital organs.

Peripheral nervous system: That portion of the nervous system other than that of the brain and spinal cord.

Peyronie's disease: A disease characterized by a deformation or bending of the penis which may make vaginal penetration impossible or painful. The disease is caused by a buildup of plaque along the walls of the erectile tissues of the penis resulting in an area of scar tissue.

Phentolamine: A drug, usually used in combination with other drugs, used in penile injection therapy.

Pituitary gland: A small gland located at the base of the brain. The pituitary gland produces six hormones, which, in turn, stimulates the release of other hormones, including testosterone. An excess of pituitary hormone, prolactin, can result in erectile dysfunction.

Plaque: A concentration of fatty tissue that takes place at some point inside the body, including inside an artery. When plaque results in a blockage in the arterial blood supply to the penis, the result may be erectile dysfunction. A plaque buildup in the penis can result in Peyronie's disease.

Postage stamp test: A simple test used to measure the presence of nocturnal erections that involves the wrapping of a coil of postage stamps around the penis and observing after, a period of sleep, whether there has been a break in the stamp perforations.

Premature ejaculation: A treatable disorder in which ejaculation takes place during sexual activities well before a point desired by both partners. The condition is sometimes caused by a prostate infection.

Prescription drug: A drug that may be obtained legally only by an order issued by a licensed physician or other approved health care provider.

Priapism: A painful and undesired erection that persists for an extended period of time. Priapism is a medical emergency that requires prompt treatment.

Prolactin: A hormone secreted by the pituitary gland that stimulates the production of breast milk (lactation) in women. An excess of the hormone in men may result in impotence.

Prolonged ejaculation: Ejaculation occurring after an extended period of stimulus of the penis. The deliberate delaying of ejaculation may result in prostate congestion and pain and discomfort.

Prostaglandin E1: A smooth muscle relaxant drug used in penile injection therapy.

Prostate (prostate gland): A firm, muscular organ made up of several individual glands, located surrounding the urethra and near to the outlet of the bladder. The prostate manufactures a portion of the seminal fluid.

Prostatic fluid: The fluid produced by the prostate gland that accounts for a portion of the semen fluid that passes through the penis during ejaculation.

Prostatitis: An acute or chronic infection of the prostate caused by common coliform bacteria. May cause premature ejaculation.

Prostectomy: The removal by surgery of all or a portion of the prostate gland to treat benign prostate enlargement or prostate cancer. May result in erectile failure.

Psychotherapy: Application of the principles of psychology or behavioral science to treat a condition that does not have a physical origin or to counter the emotional consequences of a disorder of physical origin.

Pubococcygeus muscles: A muscular system located in the vicinity of the rectum. Use of Kegel exercise to strengthen these muscles may help to improve male sexual performance.

Pulse volume recording: A diagnostic method involving the recording of the fluctuation of the penile blood pressure of a patient over a period of time and comparison with the characteristic pattern of fluctuations in men not subject to erectile dysfunction.

R

Radiation therapy: A cancer treatment involving the destruction of malignant tissue by bombardment with X rays or other forms of high-energy radiation. Radiation therapy, when used to treat prostate cancer, may result in erectile dysfunction.

Recommended daily allowance (RDA): That amount of a given vitamin or mineral determined by the Food and Nutrition Board, a committee of the National Academy of Science, Washington, D.C., as sufficient "to meet the needs of practically all healthy persons." The minimum daily requirement (MDR) is the minimum quantity of a vitamin or mineral that must be ingested to prevent a dietary deficiency.

Reconstructive surgery: Surgery intended to restore proper function in some part of the body; may be used to repair defects in the vascular system serving the penis that cause impotence.

REM sleep: A period during sleep characterized by rapid eye movements. Dreams and nocturnal erections are believed to occur during periods of REM sleep.

Resolution stage: The period following ejaculation in which an erection is lost and the penis returns to its normal flaccid state.

Retrograde ejaculation: Ejaculation that occurs without the normal flow of seminal fluid out of the body from the penis. Normal sensations of orgasm may occur during retrograde ejaculation. The condition may be a side effect of prostate surgery.

S

Scrotum: The pouch of skin, external to the body, enclosing the testicles and the epididymis.

Self-contained penile implant: A penile implant in which the entire hydraulic mechanism is located within the body of the device and, hence when surgically installed, entirely within the penis.

Semen (or seminal fluid): A cloudy, white fluid that serves as the vehicle for the transport of sperm. Semen is produced from fluids supplied by the testicles, seminal vesicles, and prostate.

Seminal vesicles: Two glands, located in the vicinity of the prostate, that supply a portion of the seminal fluid.

Semirigid malleable penile implant: A simple type of penile implant consisting of a rigid, but bendable, structure that can be surgically installed inside the penis. The implant, while in the straight position, provides sufficient rigidity for vaginal penetration. It can be bent downward at other times, although there is always some permanent rigidity of the penis.

Sensate focus exercises: A series of exercises involving male and female sexual partners designed to improve sexual performance. The exercises typically commence with simple touching and gradually progress to more erotic behavior and eventually sexual intercourse.

Sex therapy: The treatment of sexual dysfunction by the application of the principles of psychology and behavioral science. A wide variety of sex therapy approaches exists. Sex therapists also differ widely in professional training and background.

Sickle-cell anemia: A generic blood disease occurring most often among individuals of African, Mediterranean, Arabic, and Indian descent. The disease is characterized by abnormal blood flow and may result in episodes of priapism.

Side effect: An undesired condition resulting from the taking of a medication or being subjected to some other form of medical treatment. Erectile failure has been found to be a side effect of many drugs.

Smooth muscles: Muscles over which there is no voluntary control. The relation of the smooth muscle tissue of the penis is an essential element in the erectile process.

Snap gage test: A test to determine the presence of nocturnal erections that is more sophisticated than the simple postage stamp test, but less complicated and costly than the nocturnal penile tumescence test.

Somatic nervous system: That portion of the nervous system associated with conscious or voluntary activities.

Sperm: Small, tadpole-shaped cells produced in the testicles and transported during ejaculation by the seminal fluid. Sperm provides the male genetic contribution to reproduction.

Steal syndrome: A form of erectile dysfunction in which an individual is able to initially achieve an erection, but the erection is quickly lost while assuming or shortly after assuming the desired position for intercourse.

Stretching exercises: Exercises that involve the systematic stretching and relaxation of a muscle group. Appropriate stretching exercises may serve to improve male sexual function.

Support group: A group of individuals with a common problem who voluntarily and periodically meet to exchange information and to provide mutual comfort and support. The support groups that exist in connection with male sexual dysfunction have been a help to many men and their partners.

T

Testicles (testes): Two glands, found in men and located inside the scrotum, the principal function of which is to produce sperm, a portion of the seminal fluid, and sex hormones, including testosterone.

Testosterone: The principal male sex hormone. Most testosterone is produced by the testicles. A lesser quantity is produced by the adrenal glands. The hormone is an essential factor in the development of male sexual characteristics and sexual performance.

Three-piece inflatable penile implant: A type of penile implant consisting of two cylindrical elements that are surgically implanted inside the penis, a pump and valve mechanism that is implanted inside the scrotum, and a reservoir for hydraulic fluid that is implanted in the lower abdomen. The three-piece inflatable penile implant is the most expensive type of implant, but generally the most effective.

Trauma: Usually a physical injury to some part of the body caused by accident or as a side effect of medical treatment. Psychological trauma is an injury of an emotional nature caused by some form of psychological stress.

Tumor: A body mass resulting from the abnormal growth of cell tissue. A tumor can be either benign (noncancerous) or malignant (cancerous).

Tunica albuginea: A tough, fibrous layer of tissue that parallels the length of the penis and surrounds and protects the erectile tissue within the penis.

U

Ultrasound: A diagnostic and treatment procedure in which high-frequency sound waves are directed toward some portion of the body. A sonogram or ultrasound scan is an image produced by reflected sound waves from the internal organs under investigation. Some images may be computer enhanced.

Ureter: Two parallel tubes that transport the urine, produced by each kidney, to the bladder.

Urethra: The passageway for urine and semen that connects upstream at the base of the bladder and discharges downstream at the glans or head of the penis.

Urinalysis: A spectrum of diagnostic tests performed on a sample of a patient's urine. Urinalysis is employed in the diagnosis of prostate disorders, various types of urinary infections, diabetes, bladder and kidney cancer, and other conditions.

Urinary-genital system: The general name given to that part of the body involved in the elimination of urine and sexual activity.

Urologist: A physician specializing in the treatment of urological disorders. Urologists treat both men and women, but are sometimes referred to as the "male doctor," due to their special role in the treatment of the unique physical problems of men.

Urology: The medicine specialty dealing with the disorders of the urinary system of both men and women and disorders of the genital (sex) organs in men.

V

Vacuum device: *See* External vacuum device

Vascular surgery: Surgery performed to correct some form of defect of the blood vessels.

Vas deferens: Two parallel ducts that serve to transport semen away from each of the testicles. The vas deferens connect into a single duct in the vicinity of the prostate and urethra. This duct connects to the ejaculatory duct.

Vasectomy: The deliberate surgical severing and tying of the two vas deferens of a male with the object of achieving voluntary sterility. Vasectomy is not a cause of impotence.

Vein: A blood vessel that serves as the pathway for blood in the direction of the heart.

Vitamin: A complex organic chemical substance occurring naturally in foods or produced synthetically that are essential factors in the diet of humans and other animals. The most important vitamins in connection with male sexual function appear to be vitamins A (including beta carotene), C, and E. All these vitamins have antioxidant properties.

Z

Zinc: A mineral of a metallic nature that has been found to be an essential element in the diet of animals, including humans. The prostate gland normally contains a high concentration of zinc, leading to a belief that the mineral is an important factor in prostate health. There is still no convincing clinical evidence that megadoses of zinc can successfully treat erectile dysfunction.

INDEX